THE MASTER YOUR METABOLISM
COOKBOOK

THE
MASTER YOUR
METABOLISM

COOKBOOK

Jillian Michaels

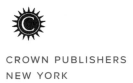

CROWN PUBLISHERS
NEW YORK

The information in this work is in no way intended as medical advice or as a substitute for medical counseling. The information should be used in conjunction with the guidance and care of your physician. Consult your physician before beginning this program as you would any weight-loss or weight-maintenance program. Your physician should be aware of all medical conditions that you may have, as well as the medications and supplements you are taking. As with any weight-loss plan, the information here should not be used by patients on dialysis or by pregnant or nursing mothers.

Library of Congress Cataloging-in-Publication Data

Michaels, Jillian.
    The master your metabolism cookbook / Jillian Michaels.—1st ed.
        p.   cm.
    Includes index.
1. Reducing diets—Recipes.   2. Weight loss—Endocrine aspects.
3. Metabolism—Regulation.   I. Title.

RM222.2.M4825 2010
641.5'635—dc22   2009053443

ISBN 978-0-307-71822-8

Printed in the United States of America

Design by Elizabeth Rendfleisch

10 9 8 7 6 5 4 3 2 1

First Edition

Acknowledgments

Many thanks to my incredible team, who work every day to help bring cost-effective, accessible life solutions to the masses:

My business partner, Giancarlo Chersich, and all the folks at NBC, CAA, Waterfront, and Crown . . . thank you!

My incredible editor, Heather Jackson; I am so lucky to have you as a friend and partner in crime.

Marah Stets, my recipe-developer-extraordinaire; I couldn't have done this without you. Thank you for your genius.

CONTENTS

the recipes

Introduction

We've all heard the famous saying from the doc behind modern medicine, Hippocrates: "Let food be your medicine." But how many people really look on their food as medicine? And how often does that medicine just not go down in any kind of enjoyable way? If you're like me, you may have spent most of your life thinking that food was your enemy. I used to think that it was simple—the more you eat, the fatter you get—so any way that could help me avoid eating calories should be exploited and explored. God, I was such an idiot. But you don't have to be.

It wasn't until I turned 30 that I realized just how wrong I had been. I found myself in the midst of adrenal burnout, which was coupled with other fun hormone-induced issues like hypothyroidism, melasma (big brown spots on my face caused by estrogen dominance), premature aging, and an *impossibly* slow metabolism. I was forced to recognize that the way I was living wasn't serving me—AT ALL—and it was time to get some answers. My quest for those answers, and what I would discover along the way, led me to write *Master Your Metabolism,* my own diet manifesto aimed at combating obesity, disease, and premature aging.

It turns out that I wasn't the only one struggling with these issues. *Master Your Metabolism* was a breakaway bestseller. Letters poured in from people all over the world who, having applied the principles in the book, were eager to share their personal success stories. But many of those letters asked for more tools to continue living a *Master*-ful lifestyle. So I felt compelled to write this cookbook and help them and you continue down the healthy path we started on together. It's imperative that the road to health and happiness be accessible to everyone, and that's what this cookbook gives you: easy, delicious recipes that allow you to be healthy in a hurry.

If you are standing in the bookstore contemplating whether or not to take this step and buy this book, consider the following: The world is becoming morbidly obese at an obscene rate. Children now have a shorter life expectancy than their parents. Cancer, heart disease, diabetes, stroke, and so on are all on the rise. We blame this devastating mess on many things, but at the end of the day it is all avoidable. Your genetics are not static. Instead, they are incredibly dynamic. The way you live and the things you eat have a DRAMATIC influence on how you live . . . and how you die. If you have the right information, you can make powerful choices that will dramatically enhance the health and happiness of you and your family.

Knowledge IS power. With this book I will educate you on which foods can greatly impact your overall health—mentally and physically—and how to make them taste great. Proper diet can prevent and control disease, give you energy, fight depression, reverse aging, and even flatten your tummy. The benefits of good nutrition are endless.

I know what you're thinking. "Jillian, the things you recommend cost money that I don't have." Or, "I am too busy to do one more thing, like cook all day!" I get it. I know those are legitimate causes for concern. That's why the Master Recipes here and the eating strategies given are designed to make healthy-in-a-hurry cooking simple and cost-effective. There are no extraneous steps or ingredients that take up time or cost crazy money. Many of these recipes are meat-free or allow you to omit meat if you're a vegetarian or just looking to save money.

Before we jump in, though, let me recap the science behind the Master Diet and Recipes so that you fully comprehend the why and how behind the lifestyle you are embracing.

the what and why

Your Biochemistry and You

....

THE KEY HORMONES

Everything that happens in your body is based on biochemistry, from your mood to your weight. And if you're scratching your head wondering just what the heck biochemistry is, I've an easy answer. It's the combination of all the molecules, enzymes, and hormones that affect and regulate your physical wellness or lack thereof.

Hormonal imbalances are frequently at the root of obesity, depression, certain forms of cancer, diabetes, high cholesterol, heart disease, gout, sleep apnea, accelerated aging—and the list goes on. The recipes in this book are designed to prevent all that scary stuff and make you hot, healthy, and happy. They optimize your biochemical potential by balancing your hormones through proper nutrition.

So getting to know the key hormones involved in weight regulation, immunity, and anti-aging is critical to your success. Let's explore the role each hormone plays in metabolic function, hunger, body fat composition, energy level, and all other aspects of general health.

Keep in mind that no hormone acts on its own. Hormone balance is like the music produced by an orchestra. If one instrument is out of tune, the whole symphony sounds like crap. The first hormone we will focus on is insulin because, as you'll see, it pops up everywhere.

We're going to crib a few pieces from *Master* to bring you up to speed quickly. If you have already read the book, it won't kill you to brush up. So start reading.

METABOLIC HORMONE 1: INSULIN

Insulin's primary function is to lower the concentration of glucose in your blood. Shortly after you eat, your meal is broken down into simple sugars and released into the bloodstream. In response, your pancreas pumps out insulin to usher blood sugar into the liver, where it is converted into glycogen for use by your muscles. When the muscles get filled up, insulin helps turn excess glucose into fatty acids and ushers them into fat cells, where they will be stored as fuel to be tapped later, if necessary. Remember, fat is nothing other than stored energy. Food, or glucose, that doesn't get utilized immediately for fuel gets stored as fat. The higher the level of glucose in the blood, the higher the level of insulin in the body.

In addition, messed-up insulin levels are related to insulin resistance (the precursor of Type 2 diabetes), heart disease, impaired glucose tolerance, metabolic syndrome, polycystic ovary disease (PCOS), kidney disease, gallstones, gestational diabetes, high blood pressure, low sex drive, gout, fatigue, skin tags, acne, and sleep apnea.

So how do we keep insulin levels balanced? Too often, the medical community thinks that "managing" the problem with drugs is the short- *and* the long-term solution. While such an approach may be an effective short-term aid to bring things under control, it fails to address the need to *reverse and eliminate* the most frequent underlying cause of chronically high insulin: *poor diet.*

The key to managing insulin is in knowing what not to eat. Maintaining low insulin levels is a key component of the Master Diet, because the less insulin you have, the more easily your body will tap that stored fat for fuel. Certain foods such as processed grains or refined sugars accelerate and increase insulin release because they have no fiber to slow down the digestive process. For this reason the Master Diet and the Master Recipes have *no* processed grains or refined sugars, and all the recipes are very high in soluble and insoluble fiber to help balance insulin levels.

METABOLIC HORMONE 2: THYROID HORMONE

Thyroid hormones help control the amount of oxygen each cell uses, the rate at which your body burns calories, your heart rate, fertility, digestion, body temperature, mood, and memory. That's kind of a lot, right?

Your pituitary gland creates something called thyroid stimulating hormone (TSH) to kick-start your thyroid. Your thyroid then takes iodine from your blood and creates thyroxine (T4), which is inactive. The metabolic magic happens when T4 is converted to T3; T3 is the active thyroid hormone responsible for regulating all the bodily functions mentioned above. As you can see, there is a lot of room for your thyroid function to get messed up. If you are having thyroid issues, it could be that you are having trouble at any point along the way.

Anything from stress, to medication, to environmental toxins can mess up the production of healthy thyroid hormones and make you hypothyroid. However, again, the number one culprit is *poor diet*. For example, when you are not taking in enough calories, your body stops producing enough TSH, and then the thyroid can't produce enough T4. Less T4 means less T3, resulting in a slower metabolism, or hypothyroidism.

Another possibility is that many of us are becoming hypothyroid because of all the processed soy in the American diet. (Read any packaged food label—I guarantee you will see it on there somewhere.) Soy has something in it called phytic acid, which can block mineral absorption in our bodies. The enzyme necessary to convert T4 to T3 needs the mineral selenium to function properly, and the phytic acid in soy can block selenium absorption. (Only fermented soy products such as soy sauce are free of phytic acid.)

When thyroid hormones are out of balance, chemical reactions all over the body get disrupted. An underactive thyroid can pack on body fat and make you feel fatigued. Graves' disease, the most common cause of hyperthyroidism, can make your heart race; you can become intolerant to warmer temperatures, you can become grossly underweight, or you can get very tired.

People with hyperthyroid glands are sometimes given radioactive iodine, which then makes them *hypo*thyroid. So you can see that thyroid balance is really tricky, with unpleasant effects at both ends of the spectrum. That's why it's important to eat in a way that protects your thyroid. If you already have a thyroid condition, eating right will help significantly, but it's very important that you consult a good endocrinologist to monitor your levels and help keep them balanced.

The Master Diet and Recipes have eliminated all of the environmental and nutritional toxins that have been shown to create thyroid problems. Even though I removed them from the recipes, here are the things to look for when you aren't cooking from the book:

- Avoid soy and foods with goitrogenic effects (swelling of the thyroid gland), such as millet, peaches, strawberries, pine nuts, bamboo shoots, and peanuts.
- Be sure to cook all your cruciferous vegetables, such as broccoli, cauliflower, brus-

sels sprouts, kale, bok choy, turnips, rutabagas, and collard greens. When eaten raw, these vegetables have high levels of isothiocyanates, which disrupt normal cellular communications in the thyroid. Cooking them deactivates roughly two-thirds of these substances in the food. Here is the catch: isothiocyanates are powerful anti-oxidants that fight cancer, so you want to be sure not to cut these veggies out altogether. Cooking them should solve your problem; if you already have a thyroid condition, eat them in extreme moderation.

On the opposite end of the spectrum, the following are power nutrients that restore and ramp up your thyroid for optimal function:

- Foods with omega-3s and iodine, such as deep-sea fish like salmon, herring, anchovies, sardines, and squid.
- Foods with selenium, such as Brazil nuts and whole grains, which help convert T4 into T3.
- Foods with zinc, which help stimulate the pituitary to create TSH; these include beef, lamb, poultry, pork, oysters, crab, yogurt, pumpkin seeds, sesame seeds, almonds, boiled spinach, whole grains, and fortified breakfast cereals.
- Foods with monounsaturated fatty acids, including olive oil, avocados, hazelnuts, almonds, sesame seeds, and pumpkin seeds, which support thyroid function.

METABOLIC HORMONES 3 AND 4: ESTROGEN AND PROGESTERONE

Estrogen and progesterone are steroid hormones. Most people think of muscle-bound meatheads when they hear the word *steroid,* but all it means is that your body creates those hormones out of cholesterol. Men and women both produce estrogens—the three main forms are estradiol, estrone, and estriol—and progesterone.

In addition to directing a woman's entire development from childhood into adulthood, estrogen has a major impact on her blood fats, digestive enzymes, water and salt balance, bone density, heart function, memory, and many other functions. Estrogen's buddy, progesterone, plays a big part in protecting a woman's pregnancy and promoting breast-feeding. Progesterone also serves as a precursor to cortisol, testosterone, and estrogen.

In women, estradiol is the estrogen of youth; in proper levels, it primarily helps a woman's body stay lean. Estradiol lowers insulin and blood pressure levels, raises HDL cholesterol, and lowers LDL cholesterol. Women with more estradiol tend to have higher levels of muscle and lower levels of fat. Estradiol also helps regulate hunger by creating the same satisfied feeling as that which comes from serotonin. Similarly, it helps keep a woman's moods stable and energy high, so she's more motivated to exercise. Estradiol does put fat on her hips and butt, but that fat can actually help her insulin response.

As a woman prepares to go through menopause, her ovaries start to shut down and her production of estradiol decreases. Then, estrone becomes her main estrogen, which really sucks. Estrone immediately shifts fat from the butt and hips to the belly. As a woman loses more of her ovarian estrogen, her body becomes desperate to hang on to other estrogen-making areas of the body, including fat, making it harder to lose that belly fat. And the more fat a woman has, the more estrone she'll produce, because fat tissue turns fat-burning androgens into fat-storing estrone. Most women tend to gain several pounds during this transition, ramping up what becomes a vicious cycle: more estrone, more fat on the belly; more fat on the belly, more estrone.

Another of estrogen's vicious cycles concerns insulin. Insulin increases the circulating levels of estrogen, and estrone causes insulin resistance. According to the Mayo Clinic, estrogen levels are 50 to 100 times higher in postmenopausal women who are overweight than in those who are thinner, which may account for the 20 percent greater risk of cancer (especially breast cancer) among heavier older women.

Progesterone helps to balance the estrogen and can help manage some of these issues, so when progesterone levels drop, that creates problems, too. For example, when progesterone drops right before a woman's period, that imbalance may trigger cravings to eat, primarily carbs. Progesterone drops again even more dramatically than estrogen at menopause. Because progesterone is also the precursor for testosterone and estradiol, when a woman's progesterone production falls off, she also starts to lose the fat-burning effects of those metabolically positive hormones. Stress can make this imbalance worse. Cortisol and progesterone compete for the same receptors on the cells, so when a woman overproduces cortisol, that threatens her healthy progesterone activity.

Men have a small amount of natural estradiol, produced in the testes and adrenals. When estrogen is at normal, healthy levels, it can help protect a man's brain, heart, and bones, as well as provide a healthy libido. When a man's estrogen is in balance with

ESTROGEN UPS AND DOWNS

People used to think that all of women's hormone-balance problems stemmed from declining levels of estrogen, especially during perimenopause and menopause, PMS, or postpartum periods. But increasingly, women in Western cultures tend to have *too much* estrogen rather than too little. In the past 50 years, doctors noticed that signs of puberty in girls—budding breasts, weight gain, pubic hair development, and menstruation—have been happening earlier and earlier. Likewise, rates of breast cancer have jumped 40 percent in the past 35 years. And decreasing sperm counts and increasing prostate cancer rates for men indicate that men are also facing problems from excessive estrogen. Men are naturally prone to increases in estrogen as they age, but any additional excess can lead to further problems with decreased metabolism, muscle building, and libido.

his testosterone, it has little negative impact on metabolism. But when the estrogen is out of balance with other hormones, a man can lose that muscle-building, fat-burning advantage. That's when men tend to develop man-boobs (affectionately known as "moobs") and love handles—features typically seen on women.

For younger men, rising levels of estrogens are almost always a product of environmental estrogens. These excess estrogens put them at higher risk of cancer, infertility, diabetes, erectile dysfunction, and other serious conditions. Phytoestrogens, such as soy and flaxseed, are plant sources of estrogen, which have a milder effect on the body.

The plan in *Master Your Metabolism* taught how to identify and remove exogenous estrogens from your diet. It helped to rebalance your life to manage the stress that can hamper proper hormone production. These Master Recipes will also show you how to remove exogenous estrogens from your diet and how to restore the whole foods, especially healthful fats, that will help your body build the right hormones to keep you healthy, skinny, younger, and happier.

Here are the things you want to avoid or consume in extreme moderation:

- Soy—steer clear of processed soy whenever possible. Fermented soy products like miso and tempeh are much better choices.
- Alcohol.
- Flaxseed—okay in moderation.

These are the foods you want to eat more of:

- Those with soluble and insoluble fiber. These are very effective in managing excess estrogen. The more fiber in your diet, the more estrogen gets soaked up and carried out with other waste. As often as possible, incorporate all-natural sources of fiber, such as fruits with edible skins, barley, beans, oats, and leafy greens.
- Foods that have high levels of plant compounds called flavonols. These help keep testosterone from being converted into estrogen. Some good choices are apples, black olives, onions, and green tea.
- Foods with indole-3-carbinol. This is an antioxidant that blocks estrogen receptors on the cell membranes, reducing the risk of breast and cervical cancers. It is found in cruciferous vegetables such as broccoli, cabbage, kale, and brussels sprouts. Just remember to eat these veggies cooked, not raw, to protect your thyroid.
- Pomegranate juice, extract, and fruit. This has been shown to block estrogenic activity by up to 80 percent and to prevent several forms of breast cancer cells from multiplying. Another study found a similar effect on prostate cancer cells. You will find this power nutrient sprinkled throughout the recipes in this book, but it is also a great snack on its own to balance your hormones and satisfy a sweet tooth.

METABOLIC HORMONES 5 AND 6: TESTOSTERONE AND DHEA

The androgens testosterone and DHEA can help you increase your energy, shed fat, and build more calorie-burning muscle. Men produce most of their testosterone in their reproductive glands. Just as estradiol does for women, testosterone helps develop a man's secondary sex characteristics, such as body and facial hair. But testosterone helps both guys *and* girls—it boosts libido, keeps energy high, protects bone, speeds metabolism, and preserves mental function in later years.

Most of a woman's testosterone comes from the adrenals, which are also the source of DHEA. A precursor to testosterone (and estradiol), DHEA may help prevent breast cancer, cardiovascular disease, impaired memory and brain function, and osteoporosis. Awesome hormone that it is, DHEA may even help us live longer.

Here is the bummer: as we age, our DHEA and testosterone levels decline unless we are mindful to preserve them with proper diet and healthy living. When we gain weight, our bodies start to convert more of our testosterone to estrogen. This estrogen can then start to overshadow the effects of the testosterone in another vicious cycle: more estrogen, more fat; more fat, more estrogen. The testosterone keeps getting crowded out of the equation.

On the other end of the spectrum, some women develop polycystic ovary disease (PCOS), a syndrome in which they have too much androgen. PCOS is intricately related to insulin resistance, but researchers are still not 100 percent sure what causes it. Women with PCOS often have irregular periods, abnormal hair growth, and trouble getting pregnant. Unfortunately, the excess androgen and the insulin resistance also send a lot of fat directly to a woman's belly, mimicking male-pattern weight gain. Because we still don't know exactly where it comes from, our best chance of avoiding PCOS is to manage our insulin levels—job number one on this diet.

Let's look at which foods to avoid and which to embrace in order to naturally boost our testosterone and DHEA. Once again, we get the big no on soy and alcohol, and a reminder to eat flaxseed only in moderation. As we already discussed, all are shown to increase estrogen, subsequently blunting testosterone and DHEA.

On the brighter side, these foods boost DHEA and testosterone, so eat up:

- Foods rich in B vitamins, which have been shown to correlate with elevated levels of testosterone. Look for grains fortified with plenty of vitamin Bs, beans, organic beef, pork, poultry, fish, shellfish, and eggs.
- Garlic and onions, which have high levels of allicin. Studies have shown that when coupled with protein, allicin can boost protein's ability to ramp up testosterone production. Allicin also inhibits cortisol (we'll discuss that next), which can interfere with testosterone's normal function.
- Niacin-rich foods, which have been shown to boost HDL (good cholesterol). This helps maintain healthy DHEA and testosterone because testosterone is created from cholesterol. This is another reason low-fat diets aren't great. We need healthy fats and good cholesterol for many health reasons, and testosterone production is one of them.
- Caffeine, which has been shown to boost testosterone levels when coupled with exercise. But remember—do *not* abuse this. Too much caffeine can release cortisol, which is exactly what we don't want; 200 to 400 mg a day is ideal.
- Zinc, which is great for boosting testosterone. The exact mechanism for this isn't known, but one study showed that supplementing zinc in older men doubled their

testosterone levels, while zinc deficiency in younger men led to a 75 percent decrease in testosterone levels. We already covered foods rich in zinc for thyroid support, but here is a quick recap: beef, lamb, poultry, pork, oysters, crab, yogurt, pumpkin seeds, sesame seeds, almonds, boiled spinach, whole grains, and fortified breakfast cereals.

• Selenium, magnesium, and chromium piccolinate—all key minerals for DHEA production. Green leafy vegetables such as spinach are good sources of magnesium. Some legumes, beans, and peas; nuts and seeds; and whole, unrefined grains are also good sources of magnesium. Brazil nuts, salmon, whole wheat, crab, and sunflower seeds are great sources of selenium. Good sources of chromium include carrots, potatoes, broccoli, whole-grain products, and molasses.

• Vitamin E, which has been shown to boost levels of DHEA in the body. Vegetable oils, nuts, green leafy vegetables, and fortified cereals are good food sources of vitamin E.

METABOLIC HORMONES 7, 8, AND 9: NOREPINEPHRINE, EPINEPHRINE, AND CORTISOL

Our fight-or-flight hormones—epinephrine, norepinephrine, and cortisol—can get us out of some pretty tight squeezes. These hormones help us make deadlines, save toddlers from tripping down stairs, and run to catch buses. But while the effects of heart-pumping epinephrine and norepinephrine are fleeting, the fat-storing cortisol's legacy is longer lasting—and deadly.

The inner part of the adrenal gland, the adrenal medulla, produces the other primary stress hormones—norepinephrine (which restricts blood vessels, increasing blood pressure) and epinephrine (which increases heart rate and blood flow to muscles). Cortisol, also called hydrocortisone, is produced in the adrenal cortex, the outer part of each adrenal gland. When we are first stressed, norepinephrine will tell our bodies to stop producing insulin so we can have plenty of fast-acting blood glucose ready. Similarly, epinephrine will relax the muscles of the stomach and intestines and decrease blood flow to these organs. (Your body figures it would rather focus on saving your life than on digesting your food.) These two actions cause some of the high blood sugar and stomach problems associated with stress.

MASTER YOUR NUTRIENT INTAKE

Bioavailability is a big word that is rather simple in its meaning: the nutrients that your body is able to absorb from your food. The vitamin value of a food is not solely determined by the total amount of vitamins it contains, but also by their bioavailability. This bioavailability is influenced by numerous factors, including how the food is harvested, prepared, and stored, and even which other foods it is combined with. The *Master* cookbook has been created so that you can get the maximum health benefits from your food. I mean, really, what's the point of eating carrots if you aren't getting their health benefits?

Here are a few tips that illustrate how bioavailability works:

- *Vitamin C* helps the body absorb non-heme (plant-based) iron. If you are a vegetarian and you are slightly anemic, some spinach sautéed with lemon juice can help—or throw some mandarin orange slices in with your next spinach salad.

- *Tomatoes and broccoli* have more powerful cancer-fighting qualities when eaten together than when consumed individually.

- Many nutrients are *fat soluble* (better absorbed by the body when consumed with healthy fats), so be sure to consume vegetables with a bit of healthy fat, like olive oil, for maximum absorption of protective phytochemicals.

- Consuming *organic yogurt* or a probiotic supplement can help improve the bioavailability of vitamin B, calcium, zinc, copper, magnesium, and phosphorous.

- Don't steam your veggies. Many *water-soluble* nutrients get lost in the cooking process. Instead, try sautéing, grilling, baking, or even microwaving.

- *Vitamin D* helps the body absorb calcium, so be sure to buy dairy products fortified with vitamin D. Many brands of coconut milk also have vitamin D added to them. Or if the process of fortification worries you, you can have a calcium-rich food and then catch a bit of sun.

- *Vinegar* in sushi rice can reduce the food's glycemic load by up to 35 percent, limiting the rice's effect on your blood sugar. This is why a small 3- or 4-ounce glass of white wine has been shown to lower insulin levels in the body, rather than spike them.

- Apply heat to *tomatoes.* Tomatoes contain lycopene, a potent antioxidant that combats aging, stroke, and heart disease. Cooking or canning tomatoes, or using tomato paste, can increase the bioavailability of lycopene by up to 500 percent.

- Grill with *rosemary.* The high heat of grilling activates cancer-causing compounds (HCAs) in ground beef and other meats. A 2005 study at Kansas State University found that adding rosemary to grilled meats can reduce HCA formation by up to 80 percent.

- Want a delicious end to your dinner? Serve a *fruit salad*. The phytochemical quercetin (found in apples and berries) works together with catechin (found in purple grapes) to help prevent platelet clumping.
- A few ounces of *red wine* or some grapes can help enhance the absorption of the omega-3 fats in fish and nuts.
- Avoid *soy products* that are not fermented. Nonfermented soy has a high concentration of phytic acid, which is believed to block mineral absorption in the body. I have often wondered if the reason so many Americans are becoming hypothyroid is in part because of all the soy in our processed foods. Don't forget, the thyroid needs iodine, zinc, and selenium to function properly. That's another reason to keep the probiotic tip referenced above in mind.

Once the stressor has passed, cortisol tells the body to stop producing these hormones and to resume digestion. But cortisol continues to have a huge impact on blood sugar, particularly on how the body uses fuel. A catabolic hormone, cortisol tells our bodies what fat, protein, or carbohydrates to burn depending on what kind of challenge we face. While the epinephrine (aka adrenaline) rush of acute stress suppresses appetite, any cortisol hanging around after the fact will stimulate it. Cortisol will increase cravings for high-fat, high-carb foods. It also lowers leptin levels and increases levels of neuropeptide Y (NPY)—shifts proven to stimulate appetite.

Once you eat, your body releases a cascade of rewarding brain chemicals that can set up an addictive relationship with food. You feel stressed, you eat. Your body releases natural opioids, you feel better. It's no coincidence that stress eaters who self-medicate with food tend to have hair-trigger epinephrine reactions and chronically high levels of cortisol. When stress continues for a long time, and cortisol levels remain high, the body actually resists weight loss. Your body thinks times are hard and you might starve, so it greedily hoards any food you eat and any fat already present on your body. Cortisol also turns adipocytes—young fat cells—into mature fat cells that stick with you forever.

Cortisol tends to take fat from healthier areas, like your butt and hips, and move it to your abdomen, where cortisol has more receptors. In the process, it turns once healthy peripheral fat into unhealthy visceral fat that increases inflammation and insulin resistance in the body. This belly fat then produces more cortisol because it has higher concentrations of a specific enzyme that converts inactive cortisone to active cortisol. The more belly fat you have, the more active cortisol will be converted by these enzymes—yet another vicious cycle created by visceral fat.

Thus, cortisol gets released by the adrenals when you are stressed, and in this day and age that happens a lot. We have irrefutable proof that such long-term activation of the stress system has a lethal effect on the body. When we abuse our adrenals as much as we tend to do, we set ourselves up for heart disease, diabetes, stroke, and other potentially fatal conditions. But before we even get there, we could completely fry our adrenals. This brings us to "adrenal fatigue." Mainstream medicine has not officially recognized the syndrome—supposedly characterized by insomnia, weight gain, depression, acne, hair loss, carb cravings, and lowered immune function—but some endocrinologists have built their practices on helping patients reverse these symptoms. If you suspect your adrenals are shot and your cortisol levels are out of whack, this nutrition plan is the perfect way to support your system in times of stress.

First, control the following:

- Processed foods, particularly refined sugars and processed grains, because high insulin levels trigger high cortisol. Restore foods high in soluble fiber—including oat bran, oatmeal, beans, bran, barley, apples, and pears—and foods high in insoluble fiber, including whole-wheat breads, wheat cereals, wheat bran, carrots, and cooked cruciferous vegetables.
- Sodium, which helps convert cortisone into cortisol. Keep salt intake to a minimum—preferably no more than 2,000 mg a day. We need some iodized salt for thyroid support, but there is way too much sodium in the American diet. Focus on reducing it whenever possible, and when you do use salt, make sure it's iodized, not kosher or sea salt.
- Alcohol. Alcohol activates the hypothalamic-pituitary-adrenal (HPA) axis, causing the adrenals to produce more cortisol. However, studies have shown that one glass of white wine a day can lower cortisol.

Increase these foods:

- Phosphatidylserine is a natural chemical that buffers overproduction of cortisol in response to physical stress. Good sources for this nutrient are mackerel, herring, eel, tuna, chicken, beans, beef, pork, whole grains, green leafy vegetables, and brown rice.
- Plant sterols and vitamin C have been shown to inhibit cortisol levels during times of physical stress. All fruits and green vegetables get the job done here. The best sources of vitamin C include green peppers, citrus fruits, tomatoes, broccoli, turnip greens and other leafy greens, sweet and white potatoes, and cantaloupe.
- Tryptophan is an amino acid that increases serotonin, lowering cortisol and enhancing your ability to deal with stress. Great sources of tryptophan are whey protein, turkey, egg whites, spinach, and crustaceans such as shrimp and crab.

METABOLIC HORMONE 10: GROWTH HORMONE

Growth hormone (sometimes called HGH) is one of the most influential anabolic hormones. It builds muscle, burns fat, enhances immunity, helps you resist heart disease, and protects your bones. Some say it even makes you happier. People with higher levels of growth hormone live longer, and better.

Growth hormone increases your muscle mass by helping your body absorb amino acids and synthesize them into muscle, and then prevents the muscle from breaking down. All these actions raise your resting metabolic rate and give you more power for your workouts.

Growth hormone is also amazing at helping you tap into your fat stores. Fat cells have growth hormone receptors that trigger your cells to break down and burn your triglycerides. Growth hormone also discourages your fat cells from absorbing or holding onto any fat floating around in your bloodstream.

Growth hormone actually counters insulin's ability to shuttle glucose into cells, nudging it into the liver instead. Unfortunately, this action is one of the reasons excess supplemental growth hormone can cause insulin resistance—which is why you have to be very careful before you decide to take growth hormone supplements.

The fact that this medically definable condition exists has given some anti-aging clinics the latitude to offer supplements to their patients interested in growth hormone's fat-burning, muscle-building traits. Just as in menopause and andropause, the sad fact is that growth hormone naturally starts to decline sometime after we reach our thirties. But we also do things that hasten that decline prematurely, and we should look to change those before we ever consider supplementation.

There are behaviors, such as sleep and exercise, that help boost HGH, but the most significant way we *suppress* our own growth hormone levels is—you guessed it—*poor diet*. When we eat too many low-quality carbs and keep our blood sugar and insulin high, it drives our HGH levels down; protein, on the other hand, can help release higher levels of growth hormone. So if we shortchange ourselves on protein in favor of carbs, we slam our production on two levels. New evidence is also starting to emerge to show that hormones from pesticides and other contaminants in our environment and diet can affect our growth hormone levels.

The Master Recipes incorporate all of the proven ways to naturally boost growth hormone.

METABOLIC HORMONE 11: LEPTIN

Scientists used to believe that fat cells were just blobs of lard waiting to get bigger or smaller. Now they know that fat is an enormous endocrine gland, actively producing and reacting to hormones. While scientists have identified many fat-cell hormones, perhaps the best studied of these hormones is leptin.

Leptin is a protein, made by fat cells, that is controlled by an influential gene called the *ob* gene. Leptin works with other hormones—thyroid, cortisol, and insulin—to help your body figure out how hungry it is, how fast it will burn off the food you eat, and if it will hang on to (or let go of) weight.

You have receptors for leptin scattered everywhere, but your brain is where this hormone is most active. When you've eaten a meal, the fat cells throughout the body release this hormone. Leptin travels to the hypothalamus—the part of the brain that helps regulate appetite—and bonds with leptin receptors there. These receptors control the production of neuropeptides, or small signaling proteins that switch the appetite on and off. One of the most well known of these neuropeptides is neuropeptide Y, which turns on the appetite and turns down the metabolic rate. Leptin switches off neuropeptide Y and switches on the appetite-suppressing signals—and the body gets the message to stop being hungry and start burning more calories. When it's working the right way, leptin also helps the body tap longer-term fat stores and thereby reduce them. But when leptin signaling doesn't work, you keep eating because you never feel as if you've had enough food.

In addition to the leptin release we get after eating, our bodies also experience a leptin surge overnight, while we sleep. This leptin surge boosts your levels of thyroid-stimulating hormone, which helps the thyroid release thyroxine (T4). But leptin can go wrong in several ways. One, you could be born with low levels of leptin. Scientists have found that a mutation of the *ob* gene hurts leptin production; this mutation causes certain children to become severely obese. Simple supplementation with leptin usually helps these children maintain a healthy weight. (This condition is extremely rare; you would *definitely* know by now if you had it.)

On the other hand, researchers are finding that many people who are overweight actually have very high levels of leptin. How is this possible? Because the more fat you have, the more leptin you produce. When the body continually cranks out excess leptin in response to overeating, the receptors for leptin start to get worn out and no longer recognize it. People with leptin resistance have high levels of circulating leptin, but their receptors cannot accept it, so neuropeptide Y never gets shut off, they remain hungry, and their metabolism slows down. (This high level of neuropeptide Y also interferes with T4 activity, further damaging your metabolism.)

Leptin resistance and insulin resistance go hand in hand, but just as with insulin resistance, if you lose a bit of weight, your body will become more sensitive to leptin and will start acting the way it was intended to: helping you push away from the table and say, "Enough!"

Counterintuitive though it may seem, our primary goal is to keep leptin levels high, especially when reducing calorie intake while dieting. Low-calorie diets can release ghrelin (see page 18) and trigger the appetite, bringing doom to weight-loss efforts. The Master Recipes use many of the following foods in order to sustain leptin levels in the body and drive down ghrelin:

- Omega-3 fatty acids can stabilize leptin levels and help the body metabolize glucose, especially if you have become leptin resistant. Look for fatty cold-water fish like salmon and herring, walnuts, olive oil, and eggs fortified with omega-3s.

- Zinc, the wonder mineral, can help to raise leptin levels. Oysters contain more zinc per serving than any other food, but red meat and poultry provide the majority of zinc in the American diet. Other good food sources include beans, nuts, certain seafood, whole grains, fortified breakfast cereals, and dairy products.

METABOLIC HORMONE 12: GHRELIN

Leptin and ghrelin act in a yin-yang way to balance hunger and satisfaction. Just as leptin tells the brain to turn off hunger, ghrelin tells the brain that you're famished.

When you're hungry, about to eat, or even just thinking about eating something delicious, your gut releases ghrelin. Acting as a messenger, ghrelin then travels up to your hypothalamus and turns on neuropeptide Y, which increases your appetite and decreases metabolic burn. Ghrelin is the reason you always feel hungry at particular moments in the day—your body's clock triggers the release of ghrelin according to a finely tuned schedule. Ghrelin levels will stay up until you've given your body enough nutrients to satisfy its needs. Because those signals can take a few minutes to kick in, eating slowly may help you eat less overall. By the time your stomach fills up, ghrelin levels start to drop again, you feel satisfied, and you can stop eating.

Interestingly, it's not ghrelin itself that makes you feel hungry—that hunger is stimulated in part by neuropeptide Y and also by the growth hormone it releases. In fact, ghrelin levels *must* rise in order to allow the release of growth hormone. That's just one of the many reasons I don't love late-night eating, especially of carbs. I want that food to be nearly out of your system by the time you head to bed because your body requires ghrelin to enable you to effectively move through all the necessary phases of sleep. Without the proper progression, you won't get to stage 4 sleep, during which you get a big pulse of growth hormone, or to REM sleep, which helps protect leptin levels.

For the rest of the day, though, the object is to keep ghrelin levels low. You don't need the extra diet-endangering hunger and all the metabolic havoc that those resulting blood-sugar ups and downs wreak on your system. You have to stay ahead of those ghrelin surges, because ghrelin is crafty about getting you to eat. New research shows that ghrelin triggers reward centers in the brain to make food look more appetizing. These areas of the brain have been linked to drug addiction for many years, and researchers believe ghrelin triggers the centers even when you don't have any reason to eat.

Constant calorie restriction keeps ghrelin levels high, which may be why some yo-yo dieters feel like their hunger just keeps getting worse the fewer calories they eat. It's all part of nature's way of getting us to eat, eat, eat. From a biochemical perspective, ghrelin is what makes maintaining weight loss so physically challenging.

Insulin and ghrelin go hand in hand, too. If insulin goes up, ghrelin levels go down. For this reason, complex carbs and whole grains are best for keeping ghrelin levels at bay. As for what to avoid, it's the usual suspects: alcohol, processed grains, refined sugar, and fried foods. Instead, choose:

- Green vegetables. These are "free," by which I mean that when you feel hungry while dieting, you can stuff yourself with these freely. Levels of ghrelin remain high until food stretches the wall of your stomach, making you feel full. High-volume, low-calorie, nutrient-dense foods reduce ghrelin levels long before you've over-eaten. All green vegetables work, especially foods with a high water content, like a light salad or vegetable soup.
- Protein. Protein has been shown to suppress ghrelin. Anything goes here as long as it's organic and you stay within your calorie allowance. A quick way to increase your protein intake is to add whey protein to any dough, batter, or smoothie.

The Power Nutrients

....

As you have noticed, there is more to this diet than just weight loss. You will eat foods that will repair, nourish, and support every cell in your body so your body works *for* you and not *against* you. Be good to your body and it will be good to you.

The following is a list of ten Power Nutrient Food Groups that you should consume foods from as often as possible—I mean it! If you'd like to look at what each one does for your body and how each helps you restore metabolic function, check out the flagship book, *Master Your Metabolism*. For now, know that these ingredients are used in abundance in the Master Recipes. Keep in mind as you read about these that the darker versions of each food group will always have more nutrients.

GO LOCO FOR LOCAL

Maybe you have heard of the local food movement, of eating local or being on the "100-mile diet." These are just ways of learning to be a *locavore:* someone who believes in producing, purchasing, and consuming locally grown foods. This movement has risen to prominence as an important part of the larger green movement. A big part of local food's environmental appeal is that it reduces or eliminates the costs, both monetary and planetary, of transportation, processing, packaging, and advertising. In addition, locally grown fruits and veggies are better for you because they are given the time to ripen naturally, allowing the nutrients that occur in the plant to mature, rather than being harvested before ripening, as is often the case with conventional produce. And chances are they are fresher and less susceptible to harmful contamination, since the food goes straight from the farm to your table. Check out page 186 for the best ways to find food grown near you.

POWER NUTRIENT FOOD GROUP 1: LEGUMES

Best Choice: Black and Red Beans

Beans have it all: protein, fiber, dozens of amazing phytochemicals, vitamins, and minerals. If you do only one thing to help you lose weight, eat more beans!

Many beans contain phytoestrogens, but unlike isoflavone-enriched processed soy products, these phytoestrogens are shown to *reduce* levels of circulating estrogen. Beans are also high in zinc and B vitamins, both proven testosterone boosters. With 8 grams of protein and 8 grams of fiber, beans and other legumes are a caloric bargain at 110 per 1/2 cup.

Check out Black Bean Chili (page 202) and Black Beans and Rice (page 210).

POWER NUTRIENT FOOD GROUP 2: THE ALLIUM FAMILY

Best Choice: Garlic

Garlic and the other alliums—onions, leeks, chives, shallots, and scallions—are incredible body detoxifiers. They stimulate the body to produce glutathione, an antioxidant that lives within each cell and fights free radicals. Glutathione's action is especially important in the liver, where it helps to remove foreign chemicals, like pharmaceuticals and other endocrine-disrupting chemicals. Other antioxidant flavonoids in onions called anthocyanins are not only incredible free-radical destroyers but also may help fight obesity and diabetes.

In addition, alliums help to lower total cholesterol—but raise "good" HDL—by decreasing the liver's synthesis of cholesterol. (Two cloves of garlic a day might be as potent as some cholesterol-lowering drugs.) Garlic also decreases blood pressure by relaxing and enlarging the blood vessels, enhancing blood flow throughout the body. Garlic, onions, and leeks also strengthen the immune system to help the body fight off foreign bacteria and fungi, common colds, and even stomach problems.

Leeks are especially cool. They have the best aspects of garlic and onions—especially manganese, a blood sugar stabilizer—plus they're high in fiber, making them a fantastic choice to keep insulin levels stable.

Cancer researchers have found that the more alliums you eat, the more protection you get from cancers of the stomach, breast, esophagus, colon, and lung. When you consider that alliums can also help stave off cognitive decline, arthritis, cataracts, and heart disease, I'd say incorporating these foods in your diet is a must.

You'll find alliums in abundance in the Master Recipes. Check out the leeks in Barley Risotto with Asparagus and Lemon (page 196); the garlic in Roasted or Grilled Vegetables with Romesco Sauce (page 180); the red onions in Thai Green Curry Barramundi (page 142); and the scallions in Fattoush Salad (page 92).

POWER NUTRIENT FOOD GROUP 3: BERRIES

Best Choice: Blueberries

I can't believe how incredible berries are for you, especially when they taste so good. The USDA found that out of a group of more than 40 fruits and vegetables, berries have the most antioxidants. Researchers found that 2/3 cup of blueberries could equal the same antioxidant power as *five* servings of some fruits and vegetables. For less than 60 calories, you absolutely can't beat that kind of nutrient density!

Berries owe their beautiful colors to anthocyanins—flavonoids that just might tip our fat-burning genes in the right direction. One Japanese researcher found that anthocyanins stop individual fat cells from getting larger and encourage fat cells to release adiponectin, a hormone that helps reduce inflammation, lower blood sugar, and reverse leptin and insulin resistance. Another study found that anthocyanins can reduce blood glucose levels after starch-rich meals, preventing insulin spikes that lead to diabetes. Combine this activity with the soluble fiber in berries, and you have a sweet treat that works hard to help you lose weight and keep your blood sugar where you want it—low. In short, berries are one of the most concentrated "foods as medicine" in our arsenal. Next time you want a sweet treat, eat some of these!

Berries for breakfast are a powerful way to start the day: try Whole-Grain Toast with Soft Cheese Spread and Raspberries (page 53), Multigrain Pancakes with Berry-Maple Syrup (page 68), or Blueberry Banana Muffins (page 62).

POWER NUTRIENT FOOD GROUP 4: MEAT, FISH, AND EGGS

Best Choice: Alaskan Wild Salmon

Salmon is an all-around nutritional rock star. High in protein, it is a rich source of selenium, which is critical to your thyroid, and vitamin D, which helps preserve muscle. But the main reason it's my preferred choice of animal protein is its very high level of omega-3 fats. Omega-3s regulate your heart rhythm, decrease blood clotting, dilate your blood vessels, decrease your blood pressure and triglycerides, and fight inflammation. You need to eat only two servings of salmon a week to cut your risk of heart disease dramatically.

The omega-3s in salmon and organic free-range meats and eggs also help manage blood sugar and fight obesity. Fish may help the body become more sensitive to leptin and less likely to become leptin resistant. Salmon is also the perfect food when you have PMS: one serving of salmon gives you a huge amount of tryptophan, the precursor to serotonin, a brain chemical associated with calm and positive moods. And eating fish also helps reduce your body's production of prostaglandins. You can blame prostaglandins for inflammation, pain, and fever in your body—and cramps. There is one huge, unavoidable bummer we have to face with fish: toxins. According to the Environmental Defense Fund (www.edf.org), many of our oceans, lakes, and rivers are contaminated with metals such as mercury, industrial chemicals such as PCBs, and pesticides such as DDT. As a result, many fish become so contaminated that the EDF recommends limited or no consumption. Were it not for these toxins, you could eat fish every day of the week and I'd be happy—and so would your hormones.

Animal proteins are also the best source of the amino acids that you need to build and repair muscle tissue; and muscle helps all your hormones work better, especially insulin and testosterone. These amino acids decrease clotting and increase blood flow; support the healthy function of your thyroid, pituitary, and adrenal glands; and regulate blood sugar levels.

You know those 25 years of trying to reduce dietary cholesterol to keep blood cholesterol levels down? Yeah, forget that. All sex steroids are created from cholesterol, so your body needs the cholesterol in meat and eggs to make that precious testosterone.

In fact, many experts now believe that there is little connection between dietary choles-terol and unhealthy blood cholesterol. Turns out, whole eggs are a nearly perfect food, with almost every essential vitamin and mineral our bodies need to function. (Pair an egg with an orange and you'll get the one thing that's missing from eggs—vitamin C.) While you need a few egg yolks to get the healthful omega-3s, cholesterol, and vi-tamins A, D, E, and K, egg whites have even more protein than egg yolks—for about one-quarter the calories. And protein increases your metabolic rate because it takes more energy to burn than carbs or fats.

You'll find here an entire chapter dedicated to meat and poultry and another dedi-cated to fish and shellfish. Plus, there are some salmon and egg recipes in other chap-ters. Try the Curried Salmon Salad Pita Pockets (page 106) for breakfast, or the Chicken Sausage with Poached Eggs and Sweet Potato Hash (page 60) any time of day!

SIX REASONS TO GO ORGANIC

No matter what causes you are passionate about, organic food pretty much affects all of them. Going organic is humanitarian because it protects farmworkers from unhealthy pesticides. If you are into animal rights, organic is a far more humane way to raise livestock. If you're an environmentalist, organic farming protects the planet because you don't have toxins running off into the soil, rivers, and oceans. And most important, organics protect *you*—you will not be eating all the hor-mones, antibiotics, pesticides, and toxins that make you fat and sick.

Surprisingly, organic food is a tough sell with Americans. No one wants to spend the money, so let's put this in perspective. How much do you think all those pre-scriptions for obesity-related diseases are going to cost? Or chemotherapy? Lots, I bet. I know people who have lost their homes because of illness. Every dollar you put into the prevention of illness will save you thousands down the road in treat-ment. Organic foods are an investment in your health, and the extra $20 a week you spend on groceries will pay off tenfold in the long run. If you still need to be convinced, here are a few other reasons to chew on.

1. **Organics help you avoid pesticides and other chemicals.** A study at the University of Washington found that the urine of kids who ate mostly conven-tional (i.e., pesticide-laden) diets had *nine times* the organophosphorus pesti-cide concentration of kids who ate mostly organic. Eww!

2.   **Organics help you prevent antibiotic resistance.** Massive use of antibiotics in the conventional meat and dairy industry leads to widespread antibiotic resistance, the kind that has made us more vulnerable to potentially fatal bacteria such as methicillin-resistant *Staphylococcus aureus,* or MRSA.

3.   **Organics taste better.** Organic produce is and will always be fresher than nonorganic produce, and fresher is better. Without pesticides and chemical preservatives, organic produce has to be eaten sooner or it will rot.

4.   **Organics make your diet more diverse.** Organic produce cannot be artificially manipulated to grow outside its natural season, so you'll switch your fruit and veggie repertoire—asparagus in the spring, tomatoes all summer, kale and sweet potatoes in the fall—and automatically get more varied phytochemicals.

5.   **Organics are more nutritious.** Organic fruits and vegetables can't rely on pesticides—they have to fight off bugs with their own "immune systems," naturally raising their antioxidant levels.

6.   **Organics help you save the earth.** Produce grown in the United States travels an average of 1,500 miles before it gets sold. But organic farming uses 30 percent less fossil fuel while it conserves water, reduces soil erosion, maintains soil quality, and removes carbon dioxide from the air.

POWER NUTRIENT FOOD GROUP 5:
COLORFUL FRUITS AND VEGETABLES

Best Choice: Tomatoes

Colorful vegetables and fruits are packed with antioxidants that fight the free radicals that cause aging and cancer—but that's just the start of their magical powers. By seeking out vegetables of varying colors you'll get a range of phytonutrients, each of which has its own particular health-promoting strengths. These colorful plant foods also happen to be incredible sources of soluble and insoluble fiber—both essential for hormone balance and impossible to get from animal products. The UCLA Center for Human Nutrition's color code system divides vegetables into several distinct color groups.

ORANGE: Foods high in beta-carotene include many orange vegetables, such as carrots, sweet potatoes, cantaloupe, and mangoes. The Vegetable Stir-Fry with Lemongrass (page 190) is one great way to get these orange veggies.

YELLOW: Most citrus foods fall into this category, and the vitamin C in citrus foods can also help us manage stress. End a meal with either Oranges with Lemon-Vanilla Yogurt Cream (page 244) or Rice Pudding (page 250), which both offer citrus double whammies.

PURPLE: We talked about some of the powerhouse purples in the berry section. Other purple fruits and vegetables, including grapes and olives, have high levels of resveratrol, a type of plant antibiotic with incredible promise for health. It can't hurt to try when both Chicken Salad with Red Grapes and Toasted Pecans (page 109) and Roasted Pork Stuffed with Artichoke, Feta, and Black Olives (page 136) are so delicious.

RED: All red fruits and veggies have the phytochemical lycopene. Lycopene is a powerful antioxidant that is believed to fight a variety of cancers, including prostate, colorectal, pancreatic, breast, lung, and endometrial. Lycopene may also help fight heart disease by halting oxidative stress, the process by which LDL particles harden and start to gunk up the arteries.

The most versatile member of this colorful vegetable and fruit list actually qualifies as *both*: the tomato. One cup of tomatoes gets you almost 60 percent of your recommended daily dose of vitamin C and 20 percent of your vitamin A, as well as plenty of vitamin K, potassium, manganese, chromium, and several important B vitamins, for just 37 calories. Tomatoes are also a very good source of fiber: 1 cup provides almost 8 percent of your daily needs and helps you counter high blood sugar.

Find your red veggies in Baked Ratatouille with Parmesan (page 204), Roasted Tomato and Black Bean Soup (page 80), or Quinoa-Stuffed Peppers (page 200).

POWER NUTRIENT FOOD GROUP 6: CRUCIFEROUS VEGETABLES

Best Choice: Broccoli

If the word *broccoli* makes you pucker your lips a little, it could be that you're a super-taster, someone who has a genetic predisposition to dislike cruciferous vegetables. But you're not getting off that easily! When you chew cruciferous veggies, you release enzymes that start the breakdown of glucosinolates, a chemical process that gives these vegetables their unbeatable cancer-fighting properties as well as their intense flavor. These compounds are the plants' own defense mechanism: by ingesting them, you take on their power.

Sulforaphane, a compound found in cruciferous vegetables such as broccoli, cabbage, and cauliflower, was recently shown to help the body repair damage brought on by diabetes-related hypoglycemia. Researchers believe these compounds can also help people prevent the heart disease that often comes with diabetes.

Don't forget our nutrient density credo: these babies pack serious nutritional power in spite of having few calories in every mouthful, primarily because of their high water and fiber content. That fiber will help fill you up and can increase your body's ability to burn fat by up to 30 percent. Studies have consistently shown that people who eat the most fiber gain the least amount of weight.

Just make sure you cook cruciferous vegetables before eating them to avoid goitrogenic effects. Try Barley with Roasted Cauliflower and Almonds (page 211) and Beef Stir-Fry with Broccoli and Shiitake Mushrooms (page 138).

POWER NUTRIENT FOOD GROUP 7: DARK GREEN LEAFY VEGETABLES

Best Choice: Spinach

More than a thousand species of plants have leaves that we can eat—but how many do we actually eat? If we could get to just five servings a day, we could cut our risk of developing diabetes by 20 percent.

That's just the beginning. Leafy greens cover the panoply of protective and healing benefits for your metabolism. Their folate—just 1/2 cup of spinach meets almost one-third of your daily needs—and vitamins B_6 and B_{12} make them huge heart-disease fighters. Greens also boast plenty of calcium and potassium, which along with magnesium help to maintain correct fluid and blood pressure levels in the body. Romaine lettuce and turnip greens are particularly high in vitamin C, which the adrenal glands release during stress.

And, of course, greens are an incredibly nutrient-dense cancer fighter. Believe it or not, leafy greens even contain a very small amount of omega-3 fats. On their own, they won't get you all the omega-3s you need, but one serving of spinach will give you half the amount in a serving of canned tuna, and even a gram of protein.

Get your greens on with No-Cream Creamed Spinach (page 220), Autumn Greens Soup (page 74), and Spinach and Red Onion Quiche (page 184).

POWER NUTRIENT FOOD GROUP 8: NUTS AND SEEDS

Best Choices: Almonds and Walnuts

When my clients are weaning themselves off of yucky trans-fat snacks, I turn them on to raw nuts, like almonds, pecans, and walnuts. Nuts and seeds hit all the right snacking notes, yet behind the scenes they're helping protect you from heart disease, diabetes, and inflammation.

There's no need to fear nuts because of their fat or calories. Research suggests that people who eat nuts twice a week are much less likely to gain weight than those who don't eat nuts.

Go nuts for walnuts in Pomegranate-Pear Salad (page 244) or for Spiced Roasted Almonds (page 236); or get your seeds with Baby Spinach with Avocado, Pomegranate, and Sunflower Seeds (page 96); or get *both* in every handful with Trail Mix (page 236).

POWER NUTRIENT FOOD GROUP 9: ORGANIC DAIRY

Best Choice: Organic Low-fat Plain Yogurt

Research is piling up that shows the calcium in dairy plays a critical role in weight control. Even small deficiencies of calcium change fat-burning signals in the cells and have a dampening effect on metabolism. But calcium doesn't just affect weight; a study of 9,000 people reported in the journal *Circulation* suggested that calcium also protects against the development of metabolic syndrome.

Grass-fed dairy products have saturated and trans fats, but they also include conjugated linoleic acids, or CLAs. Shown to improve body composition, CLAs help to drive fat out of fatty tissues, where it can be burned more easily. The combination of these healthy fats with dairy's high protein also stimulates the appetite-suppressing hormone CCK. Organic, free-range dairy tastes better, has no antibiotics or hormones, and has more omega-3s. Bonus: the zinc in dairy helps support healthy levels of appetite-suppressing leptin.

Studies on the role that probiotics play in obesity continue, but the research is clear that yogurt helps keep your probiotic numbers reinforced and strong, so you can fight off infections, inflammation, allergies, diarrhea, and even intestinal cancer—all from one satisfying and delicious food.

I frequently use yogurt, especially thick and creamy Greek yogurt, in everything from sweet to savory dishes and in marinades, dressings, and toppings. Some recipes in which it really shines are Greek Yogurt Cup with Quinoa Crunch and Berries (page 52), Creamy Cucumber and Yogurt Salad (page 214), and Almond-Orange Rainbow Trout with Chipotle Yogurt Sauce (page 158).

POWER NUTRIENT FOOD GROUP 10: WHOLE GRAINS

Best Choice: Oats and Barley

Most people don't realize that many whole grains are better sources of phytochemicals and antioxidants than some vegetables, making them even more potent in the fight against heart disease and more than a dozen different kinds of cancer. And in the end it boils down to this: the more fiber you eat, the lower your body weight and fat.

The short-chain fatty acids from whole grains may also help you eat less because they stimulate fat cells in the stomach to release leptin, the satiety hormone. The high levels of fiber in whole grains also help you feel satisfied by filling you up, slowing blood sugar release, and steadying insulin levels.

Plus, don't forget that whole grains are packed with vital nutrients—vitamin E, magnesium, iron, and many B vitamins. They've been shown to reduce blood clotting and blood pressure. They also have small amounts of plant stanols and sterols, which can help lower bad cholesterol by blocking its absorption in the intestine.

Get your whole grains in Barley Soup with Shiitake Mushrooms and Andouille (page 84) or Coconut-Ginger Yellow Rice (page 208), or try your oats two fabulous ways at two different meals: at breakfast in Steel-Cut Oats with Apples and Pecans (page 50) and for lunch or dinner in Toasted Oats and Tomato Soup (page 86).

The Diet at a Glance

....

REMOVE, RESTORE, REBALANCE

As long as you focus on three main principles—Remove the crappy foods that are killing your metabolism; Restore clean, whole foods; and Rebalance when, what, and how you eat—you can't go wrong. Another way of looking at it is to remember this mantra: Clean, whole, balanced.

CLEAN

First, you look for the dish with the smallest number of adulterating additives and hormone-disrupting chemicals.

Remove These Foods
- Hydrogenated fats
- Refined grains
- High-fructose corn syrup
- Artificial sweeteners
- Artificial coloring and preservatives
- Glutamates
- Nitrates and nitrites

Reduce These Foods
- Starchy vegetables
- Tropical, dried, and canned fruits
- Soy products

- Alcohol
- Canned foods with bisphenol-A (BPA)

WHOLE

Then, you look for foods that came from the ground or had a mother.

Restore These Foods
- Legumes
- Alliums
- Berries
- Organic meat, fish, yogurt, and eggs
- Colorful fruits and veggies
- Cruciferous veggies
- Dark green leafy veggies
- Nuts and seeds
- Dairy
- Whole grains

BALANCED

Finally, you get a healthy balance of protein, fat, carbs, and calories throughout the day.

Rebalance Your Energy
- Eat breakfast and do not skip meals
- Eat every four hours
- Do not eat after 9 P.M.
- No carbs after 7 P.M.
- Eat until you're full
- But don't stuff yourself
- Eat 40 percent carbs/30 percent fat/30 percent protein

Mastering the Health Benefits

....

CRACKING THE CODE

All of the recipes in this *Master* cookbook are designed not only to taste amazing but also to help you live your healthiest, hottest, happiest life. For that reason I have created a system to identify the amazing health benefits in each recipe—and specific foods within the recipes! At the top of each recipe, in bold text, is a list of the benefits it provides:

ANTI-CANCER

These dishes contain powerful antioxidants that help defend our bodies against free radicals and the carcinogenic damage they cause.

MASTER FOODS: practically all fruits and vegetables that are organic

HEART HEALTHY

Recipes marked heart healthy will help lower blood pressure, lower LDL (aka "bad" cholesterol), raise HDL (the "good" stuff), and fight off atherosclerosis, or hardening of the arterial walls.

MASTER FOODS: olive oil, avocado, nuts, salmon, sardines, squid, mussels, garlic, onions, and practically all fruits and vegetables

BOOSTS IMMUNITY

The nutrients in these dishes have one or more of the following benefits: antifungal, antibacterial, antiviral, and antiparasitic properties to help you fight off sickness and infection.

MASTER FOODS: garlic, chile pepper, honey, yogurt, onions

BOOSTS METABOLISM

These recipes boost metabolism by facilitating the creation of fat-burning, muscle-building hormones such as thyroid, HGH, DHEA, and testosterone while keeping stress and hunger hormones like cortisol and ghrelin at bay.

MASTER FOODS: all-natural and organic fruits and vegetables, beans, legumes, seeds, nuts (with the exception of peanuts, cashews, macadamia nuts); organic lean proteins (poultry, meat, fish), yogurts, and whole grains (amaranth, barley, brown rice, millet, bulgur, quinoa, spelt)

IMPROVES MOOD

These improve mood by managing stress, fighting depression, facilitating sleep, and inducing an overall calm by releasing serotonin and dopamine in the brain. B vitamins (especially B_6, B_9, and B_{12}) protect brain cells from oxidants, help turn glucose into energy within brain cells, and keep neurotransmitters circulating. Omega-3 fatty acids are important for health and happiness, as they help to build neuron membranes, enhance neural transmission, and increase serotonin levels.

MASTER FOODS: Vitamin B: chicken, turkey, beef, tuna, eggs, fortified cereals and grains; omega 3: salmon, herring, mackerel, white fish, walnuts, and flax

ANTI-INFLAMMATORY

The nutrients in these dishes have natural anti-inflammatory properties that help with arthritis, joint pain, rehabilitating muscle strains, and the like.

MASTER FOODS: clove, cinnamon, pineapple, ginger, turmeric, and cumin

IMPROVES DIGESTION

The ingredients in these recipes aid in digestion and help combat everything from acid reflux to dyspepsia, ulcers, and constipation.

MASTER FOODS: chili peppers, ginger, mint, papaya, pineapple, and yogurt

HEALTHY SKIN

The nutrients in these dishes contain essential fatty acids and/or powerful antioxidants to help build and maintain healthy, glowing skin.

MASTER FOODS: berries, olive oil, salmon, walnuts, and yogurt

STRONG BONES

The nutrients in these dishes contain calcium and lactoferrin, an iron-binding protein that boosts the growth and activity of osteoblasts (the cells that build bone).

MASTER FOODS: nuts (almonds, walnuts, pecans, Brazil nuts, hazelnuts) and seeds (sunflower, pumpkin, sesame), leafy greens (arugula, dandelion, endive, romaine, spinach, Swiss chard, collard greens, mustard greens, turnip greens), oysters, and yogurt

MISCELLANEOUS

These dishes contain one or more ingredients that can help with a specific health condition not listed above. To find out what these benefits are, check out the healing properties of the foods listed next.

CRACKING THE MISCELLANEOUS FOOD CODE

The foods here have many health benefits and are not limited to the benefits listed on the preceding pages. I've created this list separately, as a way to point out their additional virtues.

Apple Cider Vinegar
MASTER ACNE, ACID REFLUX/HEARTBURN, AND CONSTIPATION: Apple cider vinegar (ACV) is a natural bacteria fighter that contains numerous beneficial minerals and trace elements. This wonder food is said to help with weight loss and cholesterol management as well. It is also said to work wonders for your overall health and may even help fight diseases such as osteoporosis and cancer, memory problems, and diseases associated with aging.

Apples
MASTER ASTHMA: Apples stand out among other fruits when it comes to aiding in the general support of lung function and lung health. If you suffer from asthma, eat lots of apples!

Arame (seaweed)
MASTER LIVER FUNCTION: Seaweed naturally detoxifies the liver and aids in removing heavy metals from the body.

Artichoke
MASTER IRRITABLE BOWEL SYNDROME (ISB): Studies have shown that artichoke leaf extract helps reduce symptoms of IBS.

Asparagus

MASTER VARICOSE VEINS: Having an extra order of asparagus may help to protect against unsightly varicose veins. Why? Asparagus is a good source of a flavonoid compound called rutin. Rutin not only has anti-inflammatory properties, but also helps improve circulation and strengthen veins and tiny blood vessels known as capillaries—all of which reduce the appearance of varicosities.

Bananas

MASTER OSTEOPOROSIS: Bananas are loaded with potassium. Potassium helps suppress calcium excretion in the urine, thus minimizing the risk of kidney stones and reducing the risk of osteoporosis.

Barley

MASTER GALLSTONES: Barley is loaded with insoluble fiber, which has been shown to help prevent gallstones.

Beans

MASTER CONSTIPATION: Black beans contain insoluble fiber, which studies have shown not only helps to increase stool bulk and prevent constipation, but also helps prevent digestive disorders like IBS and diverticulosis.

Brown Rice

MASTER BLOOD PRESSURE: Brown rice is very high in magnesium, which has been shown to be helpful in reducing the severity of asthma, boosting bone strength, lowering high blood pressure, reducing the frequency of migraine headaches, and reducing the risk of heart attack and stroke.

Carrots

MASTER YOUR VISION: Carrots are loaded with beta-carotene, which is a powerful antioxidant that helps provide protection against macular degeneration and the development of senile cataracts, the leading cause of blindness in the elderly.

Chile Peppers

MASTER ULCERS: Chile peppers have a bad—and mistaken—reputation for contributing to stomach ulcers. Not only do they not cause ulcers, but they can help prevent them by killing bacteria you may have ingested, while stimulating the cells lining the stomach to secrete protective buffering juices.

Cilantro

MASTER DETOXIFICATION: Cilantro functions as a form of natural chelation therapy, helping to detox the liver and remove heavy metals from the body.

Cinnamon

MASTER TYPE 2 DIABETES: Cinnamon may significantly help people with Type 2 diabetes improve their body's ability to respond to insulin, thus normalizing blood sugar levels. Both test tube and animal studies have shown that compounds in cinnamon not only stimulate insulin receptors, but also inhibit an enzyme that inactivates them, thus significantly increasing the cells' ability to use glucose.

Cranberries

MASTER UTIs: Cranberries' powerful antibacterial properties help to fight gum disease and urinary tract infections. It is also a mild diuretic.

Cumin

MASTER DIGESTION: The health benefits of cumin for helping heal digestive disorders has been well known throughout history. It can help with flatulence, indigestion, diarrhea, nausea, morning sickness, and atomic dyspepsia. In addition, it has also been shown to support liver detoxification.

Eggplant

MASTER BRAIN POWER: A phytonutrient found in eggplant skin called nasunin is a potent antioxidant and free-radical scavenger that has been shown to protect cell membranes from damage. In animal studies, nasunin protected the lipids (fats) in brain cell membranes.

Eggs

MASTER HEALTHY HAIR: Eggs promote healthy hair and nails because of their high sulphur content and wide array of vitamins and minerals. Many people find that their hair grows faster after they've added eggs to their diet, especially if they were previously deficient in foods containing sulphur or B_{12}.

Fennel

MASTER MENSTRUAL CRAMPS: Fennel is great for many things! It has high concentrations of iron and histidine, which are helpful in the treatment of anemia. Fennel is also an emenagogue; that is, it eases cramps and helps regulate hormones responsible for menstruation. It is also a mild diuretic, aiding in detoxifying the body and protecting your liver through increased urination.

Maple Syrup

MASTER PROSTATE HEALTH: This one is for men only. It turns out that maple syrup reduces prostate size and boosts male reproductive hormones.

Mint

MASTER TUMMY ACHES: Mint is well known for its natural ability to prevent or inhibit stomachaches.

Nutmeg

MASTER KIDNEY FUNCTION: Studies have shown that nutmeg is extremely beneficial for removing toxins from the body, and even for helping dissolve kidney stones.

Papayas

MASTER MACULAR DEGENERATION: High in the antioxidant vitamins A, C, E, and in the carotenoids, papayas are great for preventing macular degeneration and promoting lung health.

Pears

MASTER A HEALTHY PREGNANCY: The high folic acid content in pears may help to prevent birth defects, as well as help keep pregnant women, and their babies, healthy.

Pepitas/Pumpkin Seeds

MASTER YOUR DEFENSES: Pepitas are one of nature's nearly perfect foods. They offer an abundance of nutrients, including amino acids, unsaturated fatty acids, and a whole bunch of minerals such as calcium, potassium, niacin, and phosphorus. They are high in most of the B vitamins, as well as in vitamins C, D, E, and K. They are also rich in the eye protective carotenoid, lutein. Snacking on just one handful of pepitas, about 1 ounce, provides a whopping 9 grams of protein, along with manganese, magnesium, phosphorous, iron, copper, and zinc.

Additionally, pepitas have recently been shown to be protective of the liver. Mice fed a mixture of pumpkin seeds and flaxseed showed a major decrease in plasma and liver toxins as well as improved efficiency of their antioxidant defense systems.

Quinoa

MASTER MIGRAINE: If you are prone to migraines, try adding quinoa to your diet. Quinoa is a good source of magnesium, a mineral that helps relax blood vessels, preventing the constriction and rebound dilation characteristic of these headaches. Increased intake of magnesium has been shown to be related to a reduced frequency of reported headache episodes. Quinoa is also a good cource of riboflavin, which is necessary for proper energy production within cells. Riboflavin (also called vitamin B_2) has been shown to help reduce the frequency of attacks in migraine sufferers, most likely by improving the energy metabolism within brain and muscle cells.

Rosemary

MASTER BLOATING: Rosemary is great for detoxifying the body, protecting your liver, and acting as a mild diuretic.

Sesame Seeds

MASTER LIVER PROTECTION: Sesame seeds contain sesamine, which is believed to protect your liver as well as to lower your blood pressure.

Shiitake Mushrooms

MASTER IMMUNITY: Mushrooms have natural antiviral and immunity-boosting properties and can be used to fight viruses, lower cholesterol, and regulate blood pressure. Lentinan, an immun-stimulant derived from shiitakes, has been used with impressive results to treat cancer, AIDS, diabetes, chronic fatigue syndrome, fibrocystic breast disease, and other conditions.

Spaghetti Squash
MASTER INFLAMMATION: Spaghetti squash is rich in beta-cryptoxanthin, which has been shown to fight inflammation in the lungs, as well as asthma and emphysema.

Yogurt
MASTER FUNGAL INFECTIONS: Yogurt and kefir contain probiotics (good bacteria) that help fight fungal infections and improve the body's ability to absorb B vitamins and minerals.

Watermelon
MASTER ENERGY: Watermelon is rich in the B vitamins necessary for energy production. Additionally, it is also high in potassium, which functions as a mild diuretic.

Menus

....

The Master Recipes in this cookbook are clean, whole, and balanced, and as long as you keep those principles in mind, you'll do fine eating any of this food (as long as you don't eat only the desserts, that is!). But I know that even when we have the best intentions—like planning a week's worth of menus at a time—life can get in the way. So I've created this seven-day menu plan to get you started. It's based on about 1,200 calories per day with a caloric ratio of 40 percent carbohydrates, 30 percent fat, and 30 percent protein.

DAY 1

Breakfast
Greek Yogurt Cup with Quinoa Crunch and Berries (page 52)

Lunch
Spinach and Red Onion Quiche (page 184)
2 cups shredded romaine with Fruit Vinaigrette (page 263)

Snack
Cheddar and Apple Slices with Cinnamon (page 230)

Dinner
Grilled Skirt Steak with Chimichurri Sauce (page 140)
microwave-steamed asparagus or green beans (page 216)

DAY 2

Breakfast
Poached Eggs on Greens with Turkey Bacon (page 54)

Lunch
Laksa with Shrimp and Vegetables (page 78)
Almond-Chocolate Blondies (page 256)

Snack
Roasted Russet Fries (page 230) with Ketchup (page 268)

Dinner
Thai Green Curry Barramundi (page 142)
microwave-steamed asparagus or green beans (page 216)

DAY 3

Breakfast
Steel-Cut Oats with Apples and Pecans (page 50)

Lunch
Green Bean Salad with Shrimp (page 98)
Hard-Boiled Egg (page 259)

Snack
Trail Mix (page 236)

Dinner
Almond-Crusted Chicken Breasts (page 112)
No-Cream Creamed Spinach (page 220)

DAY 4

Breakfast
Denver Omelet (page 58)

Lunch
Chicken Salad with Red Grapes and Toasted Pecans Sandwich (page 109)
Pomegranate-Pear Salad (page 244)

Snack
Spiced Roasted Almonds (page 236)

Dinner
Baby Spinach with Avocado, Pomegranate, and Sunflower Seeds (page 96)
Broiled Tilapia with Fresh Herbs, Mushrooms, and Tomatoes (page 146)

DAY 5

Breakfast
Pumpkin Cranberry Muffins (page 64)

Lunch
Mediterranean Tuna Salad Rolls (page 107)

Snack
Açai Berry and Pomegranate Smoothie (page 226)

Dinner
Mediterranean Lamb Burgers (page 132)
Creamy Cucumber and Yogurt Salad (page 214)

DAY 6

Breakfast
Chicken Sausage with Poached Eggs and Sweet Potato Hash (page 60)

Lunch
Tomato, Avocado, and Cheddar Burrito (page 102)

Snack
1 ounce raw almonds

Dinner
Pecan-Crusted Catfish with Cranberry-Maple Compote (page 156)

DAY 7

Breakfast
Oatmeal Chocolate Chip Muffins (page 66)

Lunch
Healthy Cobb Salad (page 100)
Chocolate-Cinnamon Frozen Banana Pops (page 242)

Snack
Guacamole (page 233)
Baked Garlic Pita Chips (page 231)

Dinner
Roasted Salmon with Pepita and Cumin Seed Crust (page 150)
Smashed Sweet Potatoes with Coconut Milk (page 223)

A Note About the Nutritional Analyses of Recipes

The nutritional information in each recipe is per serving. When a recipe serves a range, the analysis is based on the first suggested number. For example, if a recipe's yield states that it serves 4 to 6, the analysis is based on the recipe serving 4. Unless garnishes are listed in the title or are an integral part of the recipe, they are not included in the analysis.

the recipes

breakfast

. . . .

STEEL-CUT OATS WITH APPLES AND PECANS

GREEK YOGURT CUP WITH QUINOA CRUNCH AND BERRIES

WHOLE-GRAIN TOAST WITH SOFT CHEESE SPREAD AND RASPBERRIES

POACHED EGGS ON GREENS WITH TURKEY BACON

DENVER OMELET

CHICKEN SAUSAGE WITH POACHED EGGS AND SWEET POTATO HASH

BLUEBERRY BANANA MUFFINS

PUMPKIN CRANBERRY MUFFINS

OATMEAL CHOCOLATE CHIP MUFFINS

MULTIGRAIN PANCAKES WITH BERRY-MAPLE SYRUP

steel-cut oats with apples and pecans

If you've never had steel-cut oats, you're in for a treat. Chewier than rolled oats (which are often labeled "old-fashioned") and with a great nutty flavor, their only drawback is that they take longer to cook than to eat! However, the quick-cooking type makes them possible on any busy morning; and as my friend and colleague Dr. John La Puma says in his book *ChefMD's Big Book of Culinary Medicine*, there is no true nutritional difference between the regular and the quick-cooking types. SERVES 4

1 cup almond milk
1 cup quick-cooking steel-cut oats
2 apples, cored and chopped into $1/2$-inch pieces
$1/2$ teaspoon ground cinnamon
$4^1/2$ teaspoons organic maple syrup, honey, or agave nectar
$1/3$ cup chopped pecans or walnuts, toasted (page 96)

In a medium saucepan, combine the almond milk, 1 cup water, and the oats. Bring to a boil over high heat. Reduce the heat to low, cover, and simmer until most of the liquid is absorbed, 10 to 12 minutes. Turn off the heat and let stand, covered, for 5 minutes.

While the oatmeal is cooking, in a small saucepan, place the apples, cinnamon, 1/2 teaspoon of the maple syrup, and 1 tablespoon water. Cook over medium heat until the apples are softened and the liquid has reduced to a syrupy consistency, 3 to 5 minutes. Stir in the pecans and cover to keep warm.

Stir the apples and nuts into the cooked and rested oatmeal. Divide among four bowls. Drizzle 1 teaspoon maple syrup over each bowl and serve.

Calories: 280.5 kcal
Fat: 10.5 g
Protein: 7.4 g
Carbohydrates: 45.2 g
Sodium: 39.7 mg

greek yogurt cup with quinoa crunch and berries

MAKES ABOUT 2 CUPS CRUNCH; 8 SERVINGS

FOR THE QUINOA CRUNCH
1 cup quinoa
$1/4$ cup flaxseed
1 tablespoon honey
1 tablespoon olive oil

FOR THE GREEK YOGURT CUP (1 SERVING)
$1/2$ cup nonfat plain Greek yogurt
2 tablespoons Quinoa Crunch
$1/2$ cup fresh blueberries, raspberries, or blackberries,
    or a mixture
$1/2$ teaspoon honey

Preheat the oven to 375°F.

Place the quinoa in a mesh strainer and rinse under cold water until the water runs clear; this is easier to discern if you place a bowl in the sink beneath the strainer. When the water in the bowl is clear, the quinoa is sufficiently rinsed. Drain the quinoa well, shaking the strainer to get out as much water as possible.

Transfer the quinoa to a medium mixing bowl. Add the flaxseed, honey, and olive oil. Use a spoon to mix until well combined. Spread the mixture in a thin layer on a rimmed baking sheet. Bake until lightly browned, 10 to 15 minutes, stirring once. Transfer the crunch to a large plate to cool. Store in an airtight container for up to 1 week.

Place the yogurt in a small serving bowl. Top with the Quinoa Crunch and the berries. Drizzle the honey over and serve.

Per serving of
Quinoa Crunch:
Calories: 131.2 kcal
Fat: 5.2 g
Protein: 3.8 g
Carbohydrates: 18.3 g
Sodium: 6.1 mg

Per serving of Greek
Yogurt Cup:
Calories: 216.9 kcal
Fat: 5.7 g
Protein: 11.8 g
Carbohydrates: 33.1 g
Sodium: 38.7 mg

Boosts Metabolism Strong Bones Boosts Immunity Improves Digestion Healthy Skin

whole-grain toast with soft cheese spread and raspberries SERVES 1

$1/2$ ounce soft goat cheese, or part-skim ricotta, at room temperature
$1^1/2$ teaspoons nonfat plain Greek yogurt
Pinch of ground black pepper
1 slice whole-grain bread
$1/3$ cup fresh raspberries
$1/2$ teaspoon honey

In a small bowl, place the goat cheese, yogurt, and pepper. Use a fork to mash and mix the cheese and yogurt together until well combined.

Toast the bread and let it cool slightly. Spread the goat cheese and yogurt mixture on the toast. Place the raspberries in a single layer on top and mash them with a fork. Drizzle with the honey and serve.

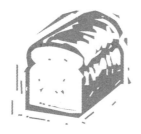

Calories: 134.0 kcal
Fat: 4.0 g
Protein: 6.1 g
Carbohydrates: 21.1 g
Sodium: 181.0 mg

MASTER YOUR SEX DRIVE

Capsaicin has been shown to improve circulation, speed blood flow, and enhance endorphin release. When you want to heat things up, *eat:* habañero, jalapeño, and cayenne peppers.

Nitric oxide is a chemical compound believed to promote sexual function in both men and women. *Eat*: organic dark chocolate with at least 60% cocoa content—have 1 ounce each day.

Zinc is known to be one of the key nutrients involved in enhancing libido and the production of sperm. Low levels of zinc have been linked to poor libido in women and low sperm count in men. *Eat:* shellfish (particularly oysters—I guess there is some truth to that advice), dark green leafy vegetables, lean red meats, and turkey.

Try Mussels with Linguine (page 166) and Chili-Lime Shrimp Skewers with Pineapple-Mint Salsa (page 170).

poached eggs on greens with turkey bacon SERVES 6

1 tablespoon any vinegar, plus 1 teaspoon sherry vinegar for the greens

6 large eggs

3 ounces nitrate-free turkey bacon (about 3 slices), cut into $^1\!/_2$-inch pieces

1$^1\!/_2$ pounds mixed tender or baby greens (such as young spinach, chard, kale, mustard, beet, or dandelion greens) or arugula, coarse stems discarded, leaves coarsely chopped and rinsed but not dried

$^1\!/_4$ teaspoon salt

$^1\!/_4$ teaspoon ground black pepper, plus freshly ground for serving

1 teaspoon fresh orange juice

Line a large plate with paper towels. Fill a large shallow pot with 2 inches of water and the 1 tablespoon vinegar. Bring to a boil, then reduce the heat so that the water is barely simmering. Crack one egg at a time into a teacup or ramekin without breaking the yolk, and gently slide the egg into the water. Poach until the whites are set and the yolks are soft to the touch, 2¹/2 to 3 minutes. Use a slotted spoon to transfer the eggs to the paper towel–lined plate and keep warm.

Meanwhile, in a large skillet, cook the bacon over medium heat, stirring frequently, until lightly browned, about 8 minutes. Use a slotted spoon to transfer the bacon to a bowl; keep warm. Do not wash the skillet.

Place the greens, with their rinse water still clinging to the leaves, in the skillet. Heat until barely wilted, 1 to 2 minutes. Do this in two or more batches, if necessary. Drain the greens to remove the excess liquid and season with the salt and pepper.

Stir the bacon into the greens, then add the orange juice and sherry vinegar. Divide the greens among six plates. Place an egg on top of each and grind some black pepper over each plate. Serve.

Calories: 175.5 kcal
Fat: 11.0 g
Protein: 13.3 g
Carbohydrates: 7.2 g
Sodium: 497.3 mg

MASTERING EGGS

Smart Selection

- Eggs often have a USDA grading system of AA, A, or B. This system represents their quality. Go with AA whenever possible. Also note that all of the recipes in this book use *large* eggs.
- Always inspect eggs first to make sure they are not cracked; cracks can lead to salmonella contamination.
- Omega-3, free-range organic eggs are the best choice, as they have all of the good nutrients and none of the bad. Studies have specifically shown them to have half the cholesterol of conventional eggs, and the cholesterol they do have is predominantly HDL.

Smart Storage

- Store eggs in the back of the refrigerator. If you store them in your refrigerator door, they will be exposed to too much warmth every time you open the fridge.
- Do not wash eggs before putting them away. It removes their protective coating, or "bloom," making them more susceptible to bacterial contamination.
- It's best to keep eggs in a sealed container so they will not lose moisture or absorb odor.
- Store eggs with the small side down. This allows the yolk to settle into the egg white, which has antibacterial properties.

- The best way to check your eggs' freshness is the water test. Drop each into a bowl of cold water. The freshest eggs are those that sink and lie on their sides; a week-old egg will tilt with the larger end up, because the air pocket inside expands as time passes, and the yolk and white have begun to separate. Week-old eggs are safe to eat and they peel easily when hard-boiled. At 2 weeks, an egg's air pocket has expanded all around the inside of the shell, and the larger end will point directly up when placed in water; if your egg floats, it's usually 3 to 4 weeks old and should be tossed out.

Smart Preparation

- Bring eggs to room temperature before hard-boiling, so the shells will crack easily after being cooked.
- It's important to cook eggs thoroughly to avoid contamination. In addition, raw egg whites contain an ingredient called avidin, which blocks the B vitamin biotin. Make sure the egg whites are not translucent, but a little yellow, and check that the yolk is not runny.
- Do not cook eggs in oil at high heat because doing so can create free radicals that are harmful to your body.

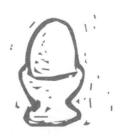

denver omelet

For a fluffy, tender omelet, make sure the whole eggs and the egg whites are at room temperature before beginning to cook. However, eggs are far easier to separate when they're cold, so separate them when cold and then let the whites come to room temperature. If you're pressed for time, place the whole eggs in a bowl of very warm water for about 5 minutes; the bowl of egg whites can be placed in a larger bowl of very warm water for 3 to 5 minutes as well.

Although many insist on using nonstick pans for omelets, a well-seasoned cast-iron skillet is a much healthier option. SERVES 2

1 tablespoon plus 1 teaspoon olive oil
$^1/_2$ cup finely chopped red onion
$^1/_2$ cup finely chopped red bell pepper
$^1/_4$ teaspoon salt
$^1/_4$ teaspoon ground black pepper
1 ounce ham, chopped (about 3 tablespoons)
2 large eggs, at room temperature
3 large egg whites, at room temperature
1 tablespoon chopped parsley leaves

Calories: 233.2 kcal
Fat: 15.5 g
Protein: 14.6 g
Carbohydrates: 8.6 g
Sodium: 579.7 mg

In a cast-iron skillet over low heat, heat the 1 teaspoon olive oil. Add the onion, bell pepper, and $^1/_8$ teaspoon each salt and pepper. Cook, stirring occasionally, until the vegetables are tender, about 5 minutes.

Stir in the ham and cook until heated through, 1 to 2 minutes. Transfer the mixture to a bowl and wipe out the skillet.

Preheat the broiler to low. Lightly beat the whole eggs and the egg whites. In the cast-iron skillet, heat the remaining 1 tablespoon olive oil over medium heat until hot but not smoking. Swirl the pan to make sure the oil fully coats the bottom of the pan as well as about 1/2 inch up the sides.

Add the eggs, onion and bell pepper mixture, and remaining salt and pepper to the pan. With a wooden spoon, mix the ingredients in the pan, making sure that the onion and bell pepper mixture is evenly spread across the pan. Cook for 2 minutes, until the bottom is set. Place the pan under the broiler and cook until firm on top, about 1 minute.

Let stand a minute. Slice into four wedges and use a thin-bladed spatula to place 2 wedges on each of two plates, overlapping them slightly. Sprinkle the chopped parsley over each and serve.

MASTER YOUR COOKWARE

Studies have shown that the chemicals in certain cookware can leach into the food you are cooking. Teflon pans, for example, have a chemical called perfluorooctanoic acid, or PFOA. This chemical may be related to liver and thyroid damage, as well as an impaired immune system.

Don't fret yet. There are healthy nonstick alternatives out there. The best are cast iron and enameled cast-iron (such as Le Creuset brand); they are stick resistant and distribute heat well. You can also use anodized aluminum. It does not react with the foods being cooked in it, plus it's nonstick and distributes heat well. Other good nontoxic cookware choices are stainless, copper-lined stainless, and copper with an aluminum core. Although these latter choices are not nonstick, they retain their heat well and conserve energy. Last but not least, you can use porcelain or glass cooking pans.

chicken sausage with poached eggs and sweet potato hash SERVES 6

1 tablespoon any vinegar

6 large eggs

1 1/2 pounds unpeeled sweet potatoes, cut into
    1/2-inch cubes

1 tablespoon plus 1 teaspoon olive oil

1 cup thinly sliced red onion

1/4 teaspoon salt

1/2 teaspoon ground black pepper

1 large Granny Smith apple, peeled, cored, and cut into
    1/2-inch cubes

1/2 teaspoon ground cinnamon

1 teaspoon maple syrup

1 (11-ounce) package chicken apple sausage links

Line a large plate with paper towels. Fill a large shallow pot with 2 inches of water and the vinegar. Bring to a boil, then reduce the heat so that the water is barely simmering. Crack one egg at a time into a teacup or ramekin without breaking the yolk, and gently slide the egg into the water. Poach until the whites are set and the yolks are soft to the touch, 2 1/2 to 3 minutes. Use a slotted spoon to transfer the eggs to the paper towel–lined plate and keep warm.

Meanwhile, place the sweet potatoes in a microwave-safe bowl with a cover. Cover and microwave on high power until almost tender, about 4 minutes. Drain and set aside.

In a large skillet, heat 1 tablespoon of the olive oil over medium-high heat. Add the onion and $\frac{1}{8}$ teaspoon each salt and pepper and cook until softened, about 4 minutes. Add the apple and cook until the onion and the apple are browned, about 4 minutes. Stir in the cinnamon and cook for 30 seconds.

Stir in the sweet potatoes and spread the mixture in an even layer; press down lightly with a spatula to brown the bottoms. Cook for about 5 minutes. Drizzle with the remaining 1 teaspoon oil, the maple syrup, and the remaining $\frac{1}{8}$ teaspoon each salt and pepper. Flip the potatoes and cook until lightly browned, about 5 more minutes.

While the hash is cooking, place an oven rack 4 inches from the broiler and preheat the broiler to low.

Place the sausages on a rimmed baking sheet and broil, turning occasionally, until evenly browned, about 8 minutes. Keep them warm if the sausage is done before the hash.

To serve, divide the hash among six plates. Place a poached egg on top of each serving of hash and place a sausage alongside. Sprinkle a little black pepper on top of each dish and serve.

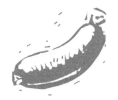

Calories: 310.8 kcal
Fat: 12.5 g
Protein: 17.7 g
Carbohydrates: 31.9 g
Sodium: 482.6 mg

blueberry banana muffins Blueberries and bananas are two nutritional powerhouses— and powerfully tasty, too! MAKES 12 MUFFINS

Olive oil spray for the tin
3/4 cup mashed very ripe bananas (about 2)
3/4 cup nonfat plain yogurt
1/2 cup honey
1/3 cup olive oil
2 teaspoons vanilla extract
2 1/2 cups white whole-wheat flour
2 teaspoons aluminum-free baking powder
1/2 teaspoon baking soda
1/2 teaspoon salt
1 generous cup fresh or frozen blueberries
1/2 cup chopped walnuts, toasted (page 96; optional)

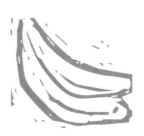

Place an oven rack in the center of the oven, then preheat the oven to 425°F. Lightly spray a 12-cup muffin tin with olive oil or line with paper liners.

In a large bowl, place the bananas, yogurt, honey, olive oil, and vanilla. Stir together until well mixed.

In a separate bowl, sift together the flour, baking powder, baking soda, and salt. Add the dry ingredients to the banana mixture and stir until just combined. Fold in the blueberries and the nuts, if using.

Spoon the batter into the prepared muffin tin. Place the tin in the oven and reduce the heat to 400°F. Bake for 35 to 40 minutes, or until tops spring back when lightly touched. Let cool in the tin for 10 to 15 minutes before transferring to a cooling rack. Serve warm. (For longer storage, let cool completely and store in an airtight container at room temperature for up to 3 days or in the freezer for up to 2 months.)

Calories: 216.0 kcal
Fat: 6.8 g
Protein: 4.5 g
Carbohydrates: 37.1 g
Sodium: 234.5 mg

MASTER YOUR SUBSTITUTIONS

- Instead of cooking with all-purpose white flour, try a variety of whole-grain or nut flours. You can replace all of the all-purpose white flour in your favorite cookie, brownie, and pancake recipes with white whole-wheat flour—flour ground from a different type of wheat than regular whole-wheat flour—which is lighter and milder tasting but has all the nutrients of the whole wheat from which it is ground. Here are some of my other favorite flours: buckwheat, coconut, whole wheat, bean, and almond.
- Instead of using refined sugar, try agave syrup, raw honey, organic maple syrup, stevia, erythritol, or xylitol. Never resort to artificial sweeteners such as sucralose, aspartame, or saccharine.
- Instead of using butter or margarine, try olive oil, canola oil, sesame oil, or virgin coconut oil.

pumpkin cranberry muffins These

delicious muffins of earthy pumpkin and warm spices are studded with tangy, antioxidant-packed cranberries and topped off with protein-rich pepitas—a perfect way to start the day! MAKES 12 MUFFINS

Olive oil spray for the tin
1 (15-ounce) can pumpkin puree
1/2 cup maple syrup
1/2 cup olive oil
1/2 cup coconut milk
1 teaspoon vanilla extract
2 3/4 cups white whole-wheat flour
1 tablespoon aluminum-free baking powder
1 teaspoon baking soda
1 teaspoon ground cinnamon
1/2 teaspoon ground ginger
1/4 teaspoon ground cloves
1/8 teaspoon grated nutmeg
1/2 teaspoon salt
1/2 cup fresh or frozen cranberries, chopped
About 2 tablespoons raw pepitas (optional)

Place an oven rack in the center of the oven, then preheat the oven to 425°F. Lightly spray a 12-cup muffin tin with olive oil or line it with paper liners.

In a large bowl, whisk together the pumpkin, maple syrup, olive oil, coconut milk, and vanilla until well combined.

In a separate bowl, sift together the flour, baking powder, baking soda, cinnamon, ginger, cloves, nutmeg, and salt. Add the dry ingredients to the pumpkin mixture and stir until just combined. Fold in the cranberries.

Spoon the mixture into the prepared muffin tin. If desired, sprinkle a few pepitas on top of each muffin. Place the tin in the oven and reduce the oven temperature to 375°F. Bake until a toothpick inserted into the center of a muffin comes out clean, 30 to 35 minutes. Let stand in the muffin tin for 5 minutes, and then unmold the muffins onto a cooling rack. Serve warm. (For longer storage, let cool completely and store in an airtight container at room temperature for up to 3 days or in the freezer for up to 2 months.)

Calories: 249.3 kcal
Fat: 12.0 g
Protein: 4.4 g
Carbohydrates: 33.5 g
Sodium: 328.2 mg

oatmeal chocolate chip muffins

These nubby muffins packed with walnuts, orange, and dark chocolate are reminiscent of fabulous German spice cookies called *Lebkuchen*. They are sweet and satisfying, so don't limit them to breakfast time. Half of one of these little powerhouses is a great alternative to crappy-for-you store-bought cookies or other junk that might tempt you during the day. MAKES 12 MUFFINS

Olive oil spray for the tin
$1^1/2$ cups white whole-wheat flour
1 cup rolled oats (not instant)
1 tablespoon aluminum-free baking powder
$^1/2$ teaspoon baking soda
$^1/2$ teaspoon salt
$^1/2$ teaspoon ground cinnamon
$^1/2$ cup coconut milk
$^1/3$ cup honey
$^1/4$ cup olive oil
1 large egg
Zest of 1 orange
1 cup finely chopped walnuts, toasted (page 96)
$^1/2$ cup 70% cocoa chocolate chips

Place an oven rack in the center of the oven, then preheat the oven to 425°F. Lightly spray a 12-cup muffin tin with olive oil or line it with paper liners.

In a large bowl, whisk together the flour, oats, baking powder, baking soda, salt, and cinnamon.

In another bowl, whisk together the coconut milk, honey, olive oil, egg, and orange zest. Add the liquid ingredients to the dry and stir just until moistened. Fold in the walnuts and chocolate chips.

Spoon the mixture into the prepared muffin tin. Place the tin in the oven and reduce the temperature to 400°F. Bake until a toothpick inserted into the center of a muffin comes out clean, 18 to 20 minutes. Let stand for 5 minutes before unmolding onto a cooling rack. Serve warm. (For longer storage, let cool completely and store in an airtight container at room temperature for up to 3 days or in the freezer for up to 2 months.)

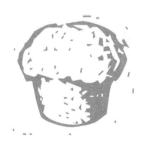

Calories: 280.9 kcal

Fat: 16.5 g

Protein: 5.7 g

Carbohydrates: 31.3 g

Sodium: 279.0 mg

multigrain pancakes with berry-maple syrup   MAKES 18 SMALL PANCAKES; SERVES 6

2 cups mixed ripe berries, such as blueberries,
    blackberries, and raspberries
$1/2$ cup maple syrup
1 cup almond milk
1 cup nonfat or low-fat plain yogurt
$1/2$ cup rolled oats (not instant)
$1^1/3$ cups white whole-wheat flour
$1/4$ cup buckwheat flour
$1/2$ teaspoon aluminum-free baking powder
$1/2$ teaspoon baking soda
1 teaspoon ground cinnamon
$1/4$ teaspoon salt
2 large eggs
2 tablespoons agave syrup, maple syrup, or honey
1 tablespoon virgin coconut oil, melted and cooled,
    plus more for the pan
1 teaspoon vanilla extract

In a small saucepan, place the berries and maple syrup and bring to a simmer over medium-low heat. Simmer until the blueberries pop, about 3 minutes. Keep warm.

In a medium bowl, whisk together the almond milk and yogurt. Add the oats and mix well. Let stand for at least 15 minutes.

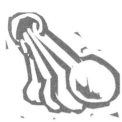

Meanwhile, in a large bowl, combine the flours, baking powder, baking soda, cinnamon, and salt.

Crack the eggs into a small bowl and lightly whisk them. Add the agave syrup, oil, and vanilla and whisk to combine. Pour this mixture into the oats mixture.

Pour the egg mixture into the flour mixture and use a wooden spoon or rubber spatula to stir together just enough to combine. Be careful not to overmix; some lumps are fine.

Preheat the oven to 175°F.

Place a cast-iron griddle or large skillet over medium heat and melt about 1 teaspoon oil. The pan is ready when a few droplets of water dropped on the surface jump and spit. If the water steams slowly, the pan is too cold, and if the water boils and evaporates immediately, the pan is too hot.

Spoon a heaping tablespoon of batter onto the griddle for each pancake. Cook for $1^1/2$ to 2 minutes, until tiny bubbles appear on the surface of the pancake and a few of them burst. Flip the pancakes and cook until browned, $1^1/2$ to 2 minutes. Place the cooked pancakes directly on a rack in the oven to keep warm. Repeat until all of the batter is cooked, using another teaspoon of coconut oil to regrease the griddle, if necessary.

Place 3 pancakes on each of six plates. Spoon the berries and syrup on top, dividing evenly among the plates. Serve.

Calories: 340.4 kcal

Fat: 8.0 g

Protein: 9.4 g

Carbohydrates: 62.0 g

Sodium: 305.4 mg

soups

GOLDEN GAZPACHO

WATERMELON SOUP WITH BLACKBERRIES AND JÍCAMA

AUTUMN GREENS SOUP

SMOOTH BEET SOUP

LAKSA WITH SHRIMP AND VEGETABLES

ROASTED TOMATO AND BLACK BEAN SOUP

LENTILS, SWEET POTATO, AND CORIANDER STEW

BARLEY SOUP WITH SHIITAKE MUSHROOMS AND ANDOUILLE

TOASTED OATS AND TOMATO SOUP

MULLIGATAWNY SOUP WITH SHREDDED CURRIED CHICKEN

golden gazpacho   SERVES 6

1 medium orange

2 pounds yellow tomatoes, cored and cut into chunks

2 yellow bell peppers, cored and cut into large chunks,
    about $1/4$ of one pepper set aside

1 small yellow onion, diced

1 garlic clove, chopped

2 to 3 tablespoons sherry vinegar

$1^1/2$ tablespoons extra-virgin olive oil

$1/4$ teaspoon salt

$1/2$ teaspoon ground white pepper

1 avocado

Using a sharp knife, preferably serrated, slice both ends off the orange. Place it upright on the cutting board and use a gentle sawing motion to cut off the rind in strips, starting at the top of the orange and following its form down to the cutting board. Chop the flesh into chunks, removing any seeds.

In the work bowl of a food processor, processing in batches, combine the orange flesh, the tomatoes, all but the reserved $1/4$ of the bell pepper, the onion, and the garlic. Process until finely pureed. Stir in 2 tablespoons of the vinegar and the olive oil. Refrigerate until well chilled, at least 2 hours.

When ready to serve, taste for seasoning. Add the salt, pepper, and more vinegar, if necessary. Halve, pit, peel, and dice the avocado. Dice the reserved yellow pepper. Divide the soup among six bowls and top each serving with a spoonful of avocado and yellow pepper. Serve.

Calories: 148.3 kcal

Fat: 9.1 g

Protein: 2.4 g

Carbohydrates: 16.7 g

Sodium: 88.9 mg

watermelon soup with blackberries and jícama SERVES 4 TO 6

5 pounds seedless watermelon on the rind
3 teaspoons extra-virgin olive oil
3 teaspoons fresh lime juice
$1/2$ teaspoon chili powder
1 cup fresh blackberries
1 cup peeled and sliced jícama, in 1-inch matchsticks
2 tablespoons chopped fresh mint

Cut the watermelon off the rind. Cut 1 cup into $1/4$-inch dice and set aside. Cut the rest of the watermelon into cubes.

In the work bowl of a food processor, place the cubed watermelon and process until smooth. Transfer the puree to a medium bowl and stir in 2 teaspoons of the olive oil, 2 teaspoons of the lime juice, and the chili powder. Let stand at room temperature for 1 hour.

Meanwhile, in a small bowl, place the reserved diced watermelon, the blackberries, jícama, and remaining 1 teaspoon each olive oil and lime juice. Stir gently and set aside.

Just before serving, stir the mint into the blackberries and jícama. Divide the soup among four to six bowls. Place a large spoonful of the blackberries and jícama on top, dividing the mixture evenly among the bowls. Serve.

Calories: 149.3 kcal
Fat: 4.2 g
Protein: 2.6 g
Carbohydrates: 29.0 g
Sodium: 4.9 mg

autumn greens soup Authentic Parmigiano-Reggiano cheese is sold in large chunks with a bit of the rind, which is always stamped with the name of the cheese. This rind is one of the hidden treasures of the kitchen, and it is well worth freezing once you've used all the cheese. Toss it in any simmering soup or broth and its flavor will permeate the dish, adding depth and a nutty taste. SERVES 6

1 tablespoon olive oil
1 bunch chard, stems chopped and leaves shredded, separated
1 small leek, thinly sliced
2 garlic cloves, sliced
$1/4$ teaspoon crushed red pepper flakes
2 small russet potatoes, unpeeled, cut into $1/4$-inch dice
4 cups low-sodium chicken broth
2 tablespoons chopped fresh oregano leaves
$1/2$ teaspoon salt
$1/4$ teaspoon ground black pepper
1 Parmigiano-Reggiano rind (optional)
1 ounce Parmigiano-Reggiano cheese, shaved with a vegetable peeler

Calories: 135.1 kcal
Fat: 5.1 g
Protein: 7.3 g
Carbohydrates: 15.5 g
Sodium: 462.9 mg

In a Dutch oven or other large heavy-bottomed pot, heat the olive oil over medium heat. Add the chard stems, leek, garlic, and red pepper flakes. Cook, stirring occasionally, until softened, about 8 minutes.

Add the chard leaves, potatoes, broth, and 4 cups water, or enough to cover the vegetables. Stir in the oregano, salt, pepper, and Parmigiano-Reggiano rind, if using.

Simmer until the potatoes are tender, 8 to 10 minutes. Remove and discard the rind. Spoon the soup into six bowls and top with cheese shavings. Serve.

FRANKEN FOODS TO AVOID

Genetically modified (GM) foods are those that have had specific changes introduced into their DNA via genetic engineering. That is, scientists take the genes from certain animals, plants, viruses, and bacteria and add them to our food. According to GM's supporters, the goal of genetic modification is to create food that is cheaper to produce, more beneficial either nutritionally or in terms of durability, or both. In other words, there might be a gene from a fish put into a tomato to make it stay fresh longer. Or scientists might engineer a pig to produce omega-3 fatty acids by introducing a round-worm gene into its DNA. Yuck!

GM foods have been around since the early 1990s. And you have probably been consuming them and are completely unaware of it. Critics have objected to GM foods on several grounds, including perceived safety issues and ecological concerns. The U.S. government does not require foods that have been genetically modified to be labeled as such. I don't know about you, but this stuff scares the hell out of me. What can you do about it? You guessed it—go organic! If I haven't scared you enough, visit www .safe-food.org to read more about these truly horrific foods.

smooth beet soup This stunning soup is not only a perfect showcase for sweet, earthy beets, it's also a nutritional powerhouse. SERVES 4

1^1/2 pounds beets (about 6 medium), trimmed and
   scrubbed
4 ounces shallots (about 4 medium), peeled and cut
   into ^{1}/2-inch slices
2 garlic cloves
1 tablespoon olive oil
1 to 2 teaspoons balsamic vinegar
^{1}/4 teaspoon salt
^{1}/4 teaspoon ground black pepper
2 tablespoons chopped walnuts, toasted (page 96)
4 teaspoons snipped fresh dill
4 teaspoons low-fat plain Greek yogurt

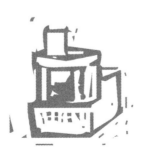

Preheat the oven to 400°F.

In a shallow baking pan, place the beets, shallots, and garlic. Pour the olive oil over the beets and stir to coat the vegetables. Cover the pan tightly with aluminum foil and roast until the beets are very tender when pierced with a thin-bladed knife, about 50 minutes.

When the beets are cool enough to handle, use a paring knife and your fingers to peel them; the skins should come off easily. Coarsely chop them and place them in the work bowl of a food processor with the shallots and garlic.

Pour 1 cup water into the pan and use a wooden spoon to scrape any browned bits from the bottom of the pan (place the pan over low heat, if necessary, to help scrape the bottom clean). Transfer the water and drippings to the food processor. Process until smooth. Transfer to a saucepan and add 2 cups water. Heat over medium heat and stir in 1 to 2 teaspoons balsamic vinegar, the salt, and the pepper.

Spoon the soup into four bowls and top each with the walnuts, dill, and yogurt. Serve.

Calories: 133.4 kcal
Fat: 6.3 g
Protein: 3.6 g
Carbohydrates: 17.4 g
Sodium: 215.6 mg

laksa with shrimp and vegetables

Laksa, whose name comes from the Persian word for "noodle," is a popular street food in Malaysia. Traditional versions of the soup are spicy, sweet, and sour and include many garnishes. This pared-down version is delicious and comes together more quickly. The laksa paste can be made ahead and kept in the refrigerator for a week or so or frozen for up to 6 months. SERVES 6

2 lemongrass stalks

3 Brazil nuts

1 fresh red chile, seeded and chopped

3 tablespoons chopped fresh ginger

2 garlic cloves, chopped

1 medium shallot, chopped

1 tablespoon olive oil

1 teaspoon turmeric

1 teaspoon ground coriander

1/8 teaspoon ground black pepper

3 ounces thin rice noodles

1 tablespoon virgin coconut oil

4 cups low-sodium chicken broth or Vegetable Broth (page 264)

1/2 cup coconut milk

1 cup diagonally cut carrots, in 1/2-inch pieces

3/4 pound large shrimp, shelled and deveined

1 cup broccoli florets

1 tablespoon Asian fish sauce (nuoc mam or nam pla)

1 cup bean sprouts

1 cup fresh cilantro leaves

1 lime, cut into wedges

Discard the tough outer leaves of the lemongrass and trim the root ends. Thinly slice the lower 6 inches of the stalks. Transfer the sliced lemongrass to the work bowl of a food processor. Add the Brazil nuts, chile, ginger, garlic, shallot, olive oil, turmeric, coriander, and pepper. Pulse until a thick paste forms.

Cook the noodles according to the package directions. Drain and set aside.

In a medium saucepan, heat the coconut oil over low heat. Add the laksa paste and cook for about 10 minutes. Stir in the broth and coconut milk and simmer for 5 minutes. Add the carrots and simmer for 15 minutes longer.

Add the shrimp and broccoli and cook for 5 minutes. Stir in the noodles and cook until warmed through, 1 to 2 minutes. Stir in the fish sauce and remove the pan from the heat.

To serve, pour the soup into six bowls and garnish each bowl with bean sprouts, cilantro leaves, and lime wedges.

Calories: 240.2 kcal
Fat: 12.0 g
Protein: 15.2 g
Carbohydrates: 18.7 g
Sodium: 464.8 mg

roasted tomato and black bean soup SERVES 4

Many food cans are laced with a toxic coating called Bisephenol-A (BPA) on the inside. Try to buy only canned food that says "BPA-free." Look for foods packed instead in glass jars (artichoke hearts, jalapeños, hearts of palm), and when buying beans and legumes, go to bulk bins or bagged options. These allow you to cut down on toxicity, save you money, and help save the environment; see soaking or cooking directions on the back of the bag. If you buy in bulk from local farmers' markets, you can obtain further preparation instructions at www.calbeans.com/beanbasics.html.

2 pounds plum tomatoes, cored and halved

2 medium carrots, sliced $1/2$ inch thick

1 large or two small parsnips, sliced $1/2$ inch thick

1 small red onion, thickly sliced

8 garlic cloves

$1^1/2$ tablespoons extra-virgin olive oil

2 to 3 cups low-sodium chicken broth, Vegetable Broth (page 264), low-sodium tomato juice, or water

3 cups cooked Black Beans (from about $1^1/4$ cups dried; page 260), or 2 (15-ounce) cans no- or low-sodium black beans, rinsed and drained

$1/2$ teaspoon dried oregano

$1/2$ teaspoon salt

$1/4$ teaspoon ground black pepper

2 teaspoons balsamic vinegar

$1/2$ cup chopped fresh basil leaves

Preheat the oven to 400°F.

Place the tomatoes, carrots, parsnips, onion, and garlic in a large bowl. Add 1 tablespoon of the olive oil and stir to coat well. Transfer the vegetables to a shallow baking dish and bake until the vegetables are softened and browned in spots, about 1 hour.

Transfer the vegetables to the work bowl of a food processor. Pour 2 cups of chicken broth into the baking dish and use a wooden spoon to scrape any browned bits from its bottom (place the pan over low heat if necessary to help scrape the bottom clean). Transfer the stock and drippings to the food processor.

Process the vegetables until smooth. Transfer the puree to a saucepan. Stir in the beans, oregano, salt, and pepper. Add up to 1 more cup of broth if necessary to thin the soup. Bring to a simmer and simmer for 15 minutes.

Stir in the vinegar, remaining $1/2$ tablespoon olive oil, and basil. Divide among four bowls and serve.

Calories: 335.5 kcal
Fat: 7.4 g
Protein: 17.3 g
Carbohydrates: 53.3 g
Sodium: 345.0 mg

lentils, sweet potato, and coriander stew SERVES 8

2 tablespoons olive oil

1 medium red onion, chopped

2 medium carrots, chopped

2 celery stalks, chopped

1 garlic clove, minced

1 teaspoon ground coriander

$1/2$ teaspoon ground cumin

1 pound dried brown lentils, picked over and rinsed

1 fresh or dried bay leaf

1 large sweet potato (about 1 pound), peeled and cut into $1/2$-inch dice

1 ($14^1/2$-ounce) can no- or low-sodium diced tomatoes

1 tablespoon fresh lemon juice, or to taste

$1/2$ cup fresh cilantro leaves, chopped

$1/2$ teaspoon salt

$1/4$ teaspoon ground black pepper

8 tablespoons plain low-fat yogurt, for serving

Calories: 301.5 kcal

Fat: 3.8 g

Protein: 17.7 g

Carbohydrates: 51.7 g

Sodium: 206.0 mg

In a large saucepan, heat the olive oil over medium heat. Add the onion, carrots, and celery. Cook, stirring occasionally, until the vegetables are softened, about 6 minutes. Add the garlic, coriander, and cumin and cook until fragrant, about 30 seconds.

Add the lentils, 7 cups water, and the bay leaf. Bring to a boil, reduce to a simmer, cover, and cook for 10 minutes. Add the potato and continue to cook, covered, until the lentils and potato are just tender, 12 to 15 minutes.

Stir in the tomatoes with their juice and cook until warmed through, about 4 minutes. Remove and discard the bay leaf. Stir in the lemon juice, cilantro, salt, and pepper. Taste and add more lemon juice if necessary. Spoon into eight bowls and top each bowl with a tablespoonful of yogurt. Serve.

MASTER YOUR HERBS

I can't imagine cooking and eating without fresh herbs. They can be added to just about every meal, from salads (throw some fresh chervil, dill, cilantro, mint, or tarragon into your bowl of salad greens) to sauces (coarsely chopped parsley, basil, and oregano add incomparable flavor and aroma to Simple Marinara Sauce, page 266) to desserts (gently torn lavender or mint leaves add depth to fruit salads).

Store bunches of fresh herbs on a shelf in the refrigerator with their stems in water—like a bouquet of flowers. Smaller bunches or loose leaves can be stored in plastic containers in the crisper drawer; if the herbs are at all damp, place them on a paper towel in the container. Herbs should not be rinsed until just before use.

To substitute dried herbs for fresh, use about a third as much dried as fresh (for example, use 1 teaspoon dried parsley in place of 1 tablespoon chopped fresh parsley). In general, fresh herbs should be added toward the end of cooking; dried herbs can be added earlier in cooking.

For more information on growing your own fresh herbs, see page 92.

barley soup with shiitake mushrooms and andouille

The immunity-boosting benefits alone are more than enough to recommend this soup, but I can't help but highlight the incredible medicinal properties of shiitake mushrooms. Not only do they have natural antiviral and immunity-boosting properties, but they also help lower cholesterol and regulate blood pressure. SERVES 4 TO 6

1 tablespoon olive oil

2 cups chopped red onions

6 garlic cloves, minced

4 ounces shiitake mushrooms, stems trimmed and discarded and caps thinly sliced

1 cup pearled barley, rinsed

4 cups low-sodium chicken broth

4 fresh thyme sprigs

1 fresh or dried bay leaf

6 ounces chicken andouille sausage, sliced

^{1}/4 teaspoon salt

^{1}/4 teaspoon ground black pepper, or to taste

1 tablespoon fresh lemon juice, or to taste

In a Dutch oven or other large heavy-bottomed pot, heat the olive oil over medium-low heat. Add the onions and garlic and cook, stirring frequently and scraping the browned bits off the bottom of the pot, until well browned and tender, about 15 minutes. Add a little water if the onions begin to overbrown.

Stir in the mushrooms and cook for 5 minutes. Add the barley and cook for 2 minutes, stirring occasionally. Add the broth, thyme sprigs, and bay leaf. Bring to a boil. Reduce the heat and simmer, partially covered, until the barley is tender, about 40 minutes. Add the sausage during the last 5 minutes of cooking.

Remove the pot from the heat and discard the thyme sprigs and bay leaf. Add water to thin the soup, if necessary. Taste for seasoning and stir in the salt, pepper, and lemon juice. Spoon into four to six bowls and serve.

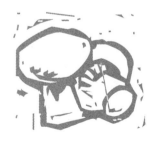

Calories: 377.4 kcal
Fat: 9.6 g
Protein: 19.6 g
Carbohydrates: 56.5 g
Sodium: 451.0 mg

toasted oats and tomato soup This soup is the quintessential comfort food: the warm, familiar flavor and texture of toasted oats complements the tangy tomatoes (use canned if ripe tomatoes are not in season), and the whole thing comes together in minutes. SERVES 4

1 cup rolled oats (not instant)
2 tablespoons olive oil
1 cup chopped red onion
3 large garlic cloves, chopped
1 teaspoon seeded and minced fresh chile
1 pound ripe tomatoes, cored and chopped, or
　　1 (14-ounce) can diced tomatoes with their juice
4 cups low-sodium chicken broth or Vegetable Broth
　　(page 264)
$1/2$ teaspoon salt
$1/4$ teaspoon ground black pepper

Calories: 240.8 kcal
Fat: 10.5 g
Protein: 9.5 g
Carbohydrates: 27.0 g
Sodium: 376.4 mg

In a large heavy-bottomed saucepan, toast the oats over medium heat, stirring frequently, until they are lightly browned and fragrant, about 5 minutes. Transfer the oats to a bowl and set aside.

Return the pan to medium heat and add the olive oil. Add the onion and cook, stirring occasionally, until softened, about 8 minutes. Stir in the garlic and chile and cook for 1 minute more. Add the oats and stir to coat them with oil. Add the tomatoes and broth and bring to a boil. Lower the heat and simmer for about 10 minutes. Stir in the salt and pepper. Spoon into four bowls and serve.

MASTERING COOKING OILS

You'll notice in these recipes that I use olive and coconut oils instead of butter, margarine, or other pressed oils. Not only are these better for your heart and health, they are among the best-tasting oils. Choose oils labeled "cold " or "expeller-" pressed. If not marked this way, the oil may have been extracted from the fruit using solvents, and those have no place in your diet.

Another important consideration when choosing oil is how strongly flavored it is. Use flavorful extra-virgin olive oil in uncooked dressings or dishes or to finish a dish at the end of cooking; it is more delicate than regular olive oil and cannot withstand high heat. Use plain olive oil when cooking or baking. Choose virgin coconut oil, which is generally minimally processed and has a wonderful flavor. The intensity of the flavor and aroma vary from brand to brand so try a variety of brands until you find one you like.

mulligatawny soup with shredded curried chicken

Use a little less curry powder than called for here if you prefer a milder soup. Red lentils cook more quickly than other types of lentils, and actually turn yellow while they cook. They are the backbone of this intensely flavorful soup. Start the rice cooking before you begin to cook the soup and everything will be ready at around the same time

SERVES 6

1 tablespoon plus $^1/_2$ teaspoon olive oil
$^1/_2$ cup chopped red onion
2 garlic cloves, finely minced
2 teaspoons grated fresh ginger
1 tablespoon plus $^1/_4$ teaspoon curry powder
Salt and ground black pepper
8 ounces dried red lentils, picked over and rinsed
1 medium carrot, chopped
1 Granny smith apple, peeled, cored, and chopped
4 cups low-sodium chicken broth or Vegetable Broth
    (page 264)
$^1/_2$ cup coconut milk
2 tablespoons fresh lime juice
8 ounces boneless, skinless chicken breast
1 cup Brown Rice, cooked (page 261)
$^1/_4$ cup chopped scallion greens, for garnish

In a large saucepan over medium heat, heat 1 tablespoon of the olive oil. Add the onion and cook, stirring occasionally, until it begins to soften, about 4 minutes. Add the garlic, ginger, 1 tablespoon of the curry powder, $1/2$ teaspoon salt, and $1/4$ teaspoon pepper. Cook, stirring, until fragrant, about 30 seconds. Add the lentils, carrot, apple, and broth. Bring to a boil, reduce the heat, and simmer, covered, until the carrot and apple are soft when pierced with a knife, 7 to 9 minutes.

Working in batches, transfer the soup to the bowl of a food processor or a blender and process until smooth. Return the soup to the pot and heat over medium heat until warmed through. Remove from the heat and stir in the coconut milk and lime juice.

Meanwhile, place the chicken breast on a work surface so that the side that had the skin is down and its underside is up. Using a sharp knife and holding it just about parallel to the work surface, start at one long edge and cut a deep incision into the meat, cutting toward the outer edge of the breast. Be very careful not to cut all the way through. Open this flap like a book. Cover the chicken with a sheet of wax paper. Using the flat side of a meat mallet, pound the breast gently to flatten it evenly. Season on both sides with $1/8$ teaspoon salt, $1/4$ teaspoon black pepper, and the remaining $1/4$ teaspoon curry powder. Brush a grill pan with the remaining $1/2$ teaspoon olive oil and heat over medium heat. Cook the chicken until done, 3 to 4 minutes per side. When it is cool enough to handle, shred the chicken with your fingers.

Divide the rice among six bowls. Spoon the soup on top, dividing it evenly among the bowls. Top each with shredded chicken and scallion greens. Serve.

Calories: 330.2 kcal
Fat: 10.3 g
Protein: 23.3 g
Carbohydrates: 37.5 g
Sodium: 122.4 mg

salads and sandwiches

....

FATTOUSH SALAD

SHRIMP AND WATERMELON SALAD

BABY SPINACH WITH AVOCADO, POMEGRANATE, AND SUNFLOWER SEEDS

GREEN BEAN SALAD WITH SHRIMP OR CHICKEN

HEALTHY COBB SALAD

RED CABBAGE AND APPLE SLAW

TOMATO, AVOCADO, AND CHEDDAR BURRITO

TOMATO SANDWICH ON GARLIC-RUBBED TOAST

CURRIED SALMON SALAD PITA POCKETS

MEDITERRANEAN TUNA SALAD ROLLS

HAM AND APPLE ON GRILLED COUNTRY BREAD

CHICKEN SALAD WITH RED GRAPES AND TOASTED PECANS

MASTER YOUR WINDOWSILL

Even if you have limited outdoor space you can utilize your windowsills to exercise your green thumb. Plant an indoor herb garden. Start with some basics, like mint, basil, oregano, rosemary, and parsley. Choose a window that gets roughly 3 to 4 hours of sunlight a day. Get planters with drainage holes in them and use soil from any nursery or garden center. Water the herbs sparingly and then use them daily in your home cooking. You'll save a ton of money—your start-up costs will be about what you'd pay for a couple of bunches of fresh herbs at the store—and you get the fabulous flavor and aroma of fresh herbs any time you want.

fattoush salad

Ground sumac, often used in Middle Eastern cooking, has a pleasantly tart and tangy flavor and a beautiful dark red color. It can be found in Middle Eastern markets or from Penzeys Spices, either at a brick-and-mortar store or online at www.penzeys.com. SERVES 4 AS A MAIN COURSE, 6 TO 8 AS A SIDE SALAD

1 English cucumber
4 cups shredded romaine leaves
1 orange or red bell pepper, cored and chopped
1 cup cherry tomatoes, halved
3 tablespoons chopped scallions (white and green parts)
2 whole-wheat pitas, toasted
$1/2$ cup fresh mint leaves, chopped
$1/2$ cup parsley leaves, chopped
2 tablespoons fresh lemon juice
1 garlic clove, crushed
1 teaspoon ground sumac
$1/4$ teaspoon salt
$1/4$ teaspoon ground black pepper
2 tablespoons extra-virgin olive oil

Cut the cucumber in half lengthwise. Use a spoon to scrape the seeds from each half. Slice each cucumber half crosswise into thin slices. Transfer the cucumber slices to a large bowl. Add to the bowl the romaine, bell pepper, cherry tomatoes, and scallions.

Tear the toasted pita into bite-size pieces and add it to the bowl with the vegetables. Add the mint and parsley. Toss with a spoon to combine the ingredients.

In a small bowl, combine the lemon juice, garlic, 1/2 teaspoon of the sumac, the salt, and the pepper. Whisking constantly, pour in the olive oil in a slow stream. Pour the dressing over the vegetables and pita, and toss gently to coat. Transfer the salad to a platter or divide among individual plates. Sprinkle with the remaining 1/2 teaspoon of sumac. Serve.

Calories: 175.3 kcal
Fat: 8.1 g
Protein: 5.3 g
Carbohydrates: 23.6 g
Sodium: 377.7 mg

shrimp and watermelon salad

Poaching shrimp in cinnamon-infused water not only adds a warm note to this sweet and succulent shellfish but also fills the kitchen with the spice's wonderful aroma. A touch of the cinnamon in the salad dressing complements the natural sweetness of both the shrimp and the watermelon. SERVES 4 AS A MAIN COURSE

2 garlic cloves, crushed with the flat side of a knife blade
1 fresh or dried bay leaf
$1^1/4$ teaspoons ground cinnamon
$^1/4$ teaspoon smoked paprika
$1^1/4$ teaspoons salt
1 pound large shrimp, shelled and deveined
$^1/3$ cup fresh orange juice
1 tablespoon cider vinegar
1 tablespoon extra-virgin olive oil
1 teaspoon honey
1 tablespoon minced shallot
5 pounds seedless watermelon, sliced from the rind and cut into bite-size cubes
$^1/2$ cup jícama, peeled and sliced in matchsticks
1 ripe avocado
2 tablespoons fresh basil leaves, torn

Fill a large saucepan with water and bring to a boil. Add the garlic, bay leaf, 1 teaspoon of the cinnamon, the smoked paprika, and 1 teaspoon of the salt. Add the shrimp, cover, and remove the pan from the heat. Let stand until the shrimp are cooked, about 15 minutes. Drain and let cool for 10 minutes, then refrigerate for 30 minutes.

Meanwhile, in a small bowl, whisk together the orange juice, vinegar, olive oil, honey, shallot, remaining 1/4 teaspoon cinnamon, and remaining 1/4 teaspoon salt. Set aside.

Place the watermelon and the jícama in a large bowl. Pour half of the dressing over and toss gently to coat. Transfer to a serving platter or individual plates.

Pit and peel the avocado and thinly slice it. Arrange the avocado slices and the shrimp on top of the watermelon. Drizzle with the remaining dressing and sprinkle the torn basil leaves on top. Serve.

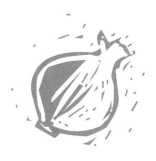

Calories: 310.6 kcal
Fat: 12.3 g
Protein: 21.2 g
Carbohydrates: 32.3 g
Sodium: 351.0 mg

HEALTH BENEFITS:

**Anti-Cancer Heart Healthy Boosts Immunity Improves Digestion Healthy Skin Boosts Metabolism
Anti-Inflammatory Miscellaneous**

TOASTING SEEDS AND NUTS

To toast on the stovetop, put the seeds or nuts in a small cast-iron or other heavy skillet over medium-high heat. Cook, shaking the pan continuously, until the seeds or nuts smell fragrant and are golden, about 2 minutes for seeds or finely chopped nuts and about 4 minutes for nuts. Immediately transfer to a plate to cool.

To toast in the oven, preheat the oven to 350°F. Spread the seeds or nuts in a single layer on a rimmed baking sheet. Toast in the oven until fragrant and lightly golden, 2 to 3 minutes for seeds and 5 to 6 minutes for nuts.

baby spinach with avocado, pomegranate, and sunflower seeds SERVES 6 TO 8 AS A SIDE SALAD

$1/2$ teaspoon grated orange zest
$1/4$ cup fresh orange juice
$1/2$ teaspoon grated lime zest
2 tablespoons fresh lime juice
1 large shallot, quartered
1 tablespoon extra-virgin olive oil
$1/4$ teaspoon chili powder
$1/4$ teaspoon salt
$1/4$ teaspoon ground black pepper
1 pomegranate
10 ounces baby spinach leaves, cleaned and patted dry
2 tablespoons sunflower seeds, toasted (see sidebar at left)
1 avocado

In a blender, combine the orange zest and juice, lime zest and juice, shallot, olive oil, chili powder, salt, and pepper. Blend until smooth. Set aside.

Fill a large bowl with cold water. Cut the pomegranate in half through the stem. Hold one pomegranate half under the water and remove the seeds with your hands. Drain the seeds well, discarding the membrane. Set aside 3/4 cup. Reserve the rest for another use.

In a large bowl, combine the spinach, all but 2 tablespoons of the pomegranate seeds, the sunflower seeds, and about 1/4 cup of the dressing. Toss gently to coat. Transfer the salad to a platter or individual plates.

Pit and peel the avocado and slice it thinly. Arrange the avocado slices on top of the salad. Sprinkle the reserved pomegranate seeds on top. Drizzle with the reserved dressing and serve.

Calories: 136.7 kcal
Fat: 8.6 g
Protein: 2.9 g
Carbohydrates: 15.5 g
Sodium: 159.2 mg

green bean salad with shrimp or chicken SERVES 4 AS A MAIN COURSE

$2^1/2$ tablespoons red wine vinegar

3 garlic cloves, finely chopped

1 tablespoon chopped fresh oregano leaves

$1/4$ teaspoon salt

$1/4$ teaspoon ground black pepper

3 tablespoons extra-virgin olive oil

$1/2$ pound shrimp, shelled and deveined, or $1/2$ pound boneless, skinless chicken breast, thinly sliced on the diagonal

1 pound green beans or a mix of yellow and green beans, trimmed

1 pint cherry tomatoes, halved

$1/4$ cup pitted kalamata olives

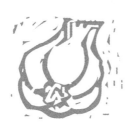

In a small bowl, whisk together the vinegar, garlic, oregano, salt, and pepper. Whisking constantly, pour in the olive oil in a steady stream. Place the shrimp or chicken in a small bowl and pour 1/4 cup of the dressing over it. Turn to coat. Cover and place in the refrigerator for 30 minutes.

Meanwhile, prepare a large bowl of ice water.

Place the beans in a microwave-safe bowl. Cover and microwave on high until the green beans are bright green and crisp-tender, about 3 minutes. Drain the beans and immediately plunge them into the ice water. Drain thoroughly.

Place a rack 4 inches from the broiler and heat the broiler on high. Spread the shrimp or chicken on a rimmed baking sheet and broil until thoroughly cooked and firm, about 3 minutes.

In a medium bowl, mix the tomatoes and olives. Add the beans and reserved dressing and toss. Transfer the beans to a serving platter or four individual plates. Arrange the shrimp or chicken on top and serve.

With shrimp:
Calories: 208.6 kcal
Fat: 13.2 g
Protein: 12.0 g
Carbohydrates: 12.3 g
Sodium: 222.9 mg

With chicken:
Calories: 226.8 kcal
Fat: 14.0 g
Protein: 14.4 g
Carbohydrates: 12.3 g
Sodium: 153.6 mg

healthy cobb salad

Cobb salad traditionally includes a good-size pile of crumbled Roquefort; delicious, to be sure, but a calorie- and sodium-buster. Here, a reasonable amount of the Roquefort is blended into a creamy dressing, so you still get the salty, tangy flavor of the cheese without overloading on the stuff.

SERVES 6 AS A MAIN COURSE

1 ounce Roquefort cheese
$1/4$ cup nonfat plain Greek yogurt
2 teaspoons red wine vinegar
$1/8$ teaspoon ground black pepper
4 slices nitrate-free turkey bacon, cut into $3/4$-inch pieces
8 cups thinly sliced romaine lettuce, rinsed
1 pound boneless, skinless chicken breast, poached (page 258) and thinly sliced
2 cups cherry tomatoes, halved
3 Hard-Boiled Eggs (page 259), peeled and quartered
1 firm, ripe avocado, pitted, peeled, and thinly sliced

Place the Roquefort, yogurt, vinegar, and pepper in a blender. Blend until smooth. Set aside.

In a cast-iron or other heavy skillet, cook the turkey bacon over medium-high heat, stirring frequently, until crisp, about 8 minutes.

While the bacon is cooking, place the lettuce on a large platter or divide it among six individual plates. When the bacon is done, pile it on top of the lettuce. Pile on top of the lettuce in neat mounds the sliced chicken, cherry tomatoes, eggs, and avocado. Drizzle with the dressing or serve it in a small dish alongside the salad.

Calories: 284.7 kcal
Fat: 16.0 g
Protein: 27.5 g
Carbohydrates: 8.7 g
Sodium: 599.7 mg

red cabbage and apple slaw This

apple-based recipe is a fun and delicious way to keep the

doctor away. SERVES 8 AS A SIDE SALAD

> $1/2$ cup distilled white vinegar
> $1/4$ cup low-fat plain Greek yogurt
> 1 teaspoon cider vinegar
> 1 teaspoon maple syrup
> $1/8$ teaspoon salt
> $1/8$ teaspoon ground black pepper
> $1/2$ head of red cabbage
> $1/2$ Granny Smith apple, cored, unpeeled, and sliced into matchsticks
> 1 small shallot, thinly sliced
> $1/3$ cup chopped walnut pieces, toasted (page 96)

Prepare a bowl of ice water. Fill a large saucepan with water. Add the distilled vinegar and bring the water to a boil.

While the water is coming to a boil, prepare the dressing. In a small bowl, combine the yogurt, cider vinegar, maple syrup, salt, and pepper. Whisk together until blended. Set aside.

Fit a food processor with its slicing disc. Cut the cabbage into wedges and push the wedges down the feeder tube to shred it. Add the cabbage to the boiling water and cook for 10 seconds. Drain and immediately plunge the cabbage into the ice water to stop the cooking. Drain thoroughly, and transfer the cabbage to a large bowl.

Add the apple, shallot, and walnuts. Pour the dressing over the slaw, and toss to coat. Refrigerate for 1 hour before serving.

Calories: 69.9 kcal

Fat: 3.5 g

Protein: 2.6 g

Carbohydrates: 9.0 g

Sodium: 46.8 mg

tomato, avocado, and cheddar burrito SERVES 4

4 (10-inch) whole-wheat tortillas
3 plum tomatoes, cored and thinly sliced
4 tablespoons thinly sliced red onion
1 ounce low-fat Cheddar cheese, grated (about 1 cup)
1 firm, ripe avocado, pitted, peeled, and thinly sliced
Freshly ground black pepper to taste
8 large basil leaves
4 cups shredded romaine lettuce

MASTERING ENERGY

Vitamin C has been shown to reduce fatigue by increasing iron absorption. It also stabilizes your energy during stressful situations by supporting your adrenal system and inhibiting the stress hormone cortisol. *Eat:* citrus—lemons, limes, grapefruits, oranges, tangerines; berries—raspberries, blueberries, blackberries; cherries; broccoli; tomatoes; kiwi; red, orange, or yellow bell peppers; and papaya.

Complex carbohydrates are high in fiber so they are absorbed more slowly, which stabilizes your blood sugar and provides you with longer-lasting energy. *Eat:* oats, quinoa, brown rice, and barley.

Choline and tyrosine are vital to the production of dopamine and norepinephrine, which improve brain function, helping you feel alert and energetic. *Eat:* organic eggs.

Vitamin B_{12} helps fight fatigue by building strong red blood cells. *Eat:* organic yogurt or kefir.

Pantothenic acid and riboflavin are needed to produce energy in our bodies. To boost energy, *eat:* sea vegetables such as arame and nori.

Position a rack 4 inches below the broiler and heat the broiler to high. Alternatively, have ready a cast-iron griddle or other heavy-bottomed pan and when ready to cook, heat it over medium-high heat.

Lay the tortillas on the work surface. Arrange the tomatoes in a straight line down the center of each tortilla, slightly overlapping them and dividing them equally among the 4 tortillas. Divide the onion among the tortillas, evenly spreading it down each row of tomatoes. Sprinkle the cheese on top of each.

Carefully slide one tortilla onto a rimless baking sheet and place under the broiler until the cheese is melted and bubbling, about 1 minute. Or transfer 1 or 2 tortillas to the griddle and heat until the cheese is melted and bubbling, about 2 minutes.

Slide the warmed tortilla onto a plate. Repeat with the remaining tortillas.

Meanwhile, top the warmed cheese with one-fourth of the avo-cado slices. Grind a little black pepper on top, if desired. Tear 2 basil leaves into small pieces and sprinkle over the vegeta-bles. Top with 1 cup of lettuce and roll up the burrito into a tight cylinder. Repeat with the remaining burritos.

Slice each burrito in half and serve.

Calories: 260.5 kcal
Fat: 11.8 g
Protein: 8.3 g
Carbohydrates: 31.3 g
Sodium: 223.7 mg

tomato sandwich on garlic-rubbed toast SERVES 4

FOOD FIGHT: LOCAL VS. ORGANIC

Why does everything have to be a fight? This seems a silly debate to me. When it comes to food, *local* and *organic* are both important. One saves you money and saves the environment (which indirectly saves you), and the other keeps you from getting poisoned. Hmmm. The good news is that it is possible to have both. Just be sure when you visit your local farmers' market to ask which vendors are organic.

1 medium carrot, grated (about 1 cup)
1 cup thinly sliced English or other thin-skinned cucumber, unpeeled, in half-moons
1/4 cup thinly sliced red onion
1/4 cup pitted kalamata olives, chopped
1 tablespoon chopped fresh oregano leaves
1 tablespoon extra-virgin olive oil
1 teaspoon red wine vinegar
1/8 teaspoon salt
1/8 teaspoon ground black pepper
8 slices crusty whole-wheat bread, such as country loaf
1 to 2 garlic cloves
1 large heirloom tomato (about 1 pound), cut in half through the stem and thinly sliced

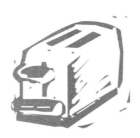

In a medium bowl, place the carrot, cucumber, onion, olives, oregano, olive oil, vinegar, salt, and pepper. Toss gently to combine. Set aside.

Position a rack 6 inches from the broiler and set the broiler on low. Place the bread directly on the rack and toast until lightly browned on each side, 1 to 2 minutes per side. Alternatively, you can use a toaster to lightly toast the bread.

Slice the garlic cloves in half. Rub the cut sides of the garlic on one side of each piece of toast. Set aside 4 pieces of toast.

Lay the remaining 4 pieces of toast on the work surface, garlic-rubbed side up. Divide the tomato slices among the 4 pieces of toast. Spoon the carrot slaw on top of each, spreading it so it covers the tomato slices. Place 1 of the reserved pieces of toast garlic-rubbed side down on top of each; use your hand to press down slightly on the top piece of toast. Slice each sandwich in half and serve.

Calories: 278.7 kcal
Fat: 7.9 g
Protein: 9.5 g
Carbohydrates: 42.5 g
Sodium: 469.3 mg

curried salmon salad pita pockets

SERVES 2

1 (6-ounce) can wild Alaskan salmon, drained
2 tablespoons low-fat plain Greek yogurt
1 tablespoon finely chopped red onion
$1/2$ teaspoon fresh lemon juice, or to taste
$1/4$ teaspoon curry powder
$1/4$ teaspoon honey
$1/8$ teaspoon salt
$1/8$ teaspoon freshly ground black pepper, or to taste
2 (6-inch) whole-wheat pitas
12 slices English cucumber (2 ounces)
2 romaine lettuce leaves, rinsed and dried

In a medium bowl, place the drained salmon, yogurt, onion, lemon juice, curry powder, honey, salt, and pepper. Use a fork to gently loosen the salmon and combine it with the other ingredients. Taste and add more lemon juice if desired.

Split the pita breads open. Divide the salmon salad between them, spreading it to cover one half of each pita. Arrange the cucumber slices on top. Grind a little more black pepper on top, if desired. Place a lettuce leaf on top of each. Replace the top of the pita and slice in half. Serve.

Calories: 264.4 kcal
Fat: 8.3 g
Protein: 22.4 g
Carbohydrates: 28.2 g
Sodium: 729.6 mg

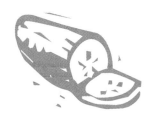

HEALTH BENEFITS:

Heart Healthy Boosts Metabolism Improves Digestion Miscellaneous

mediterranean tuna salad rolls SERVES 2

1 (6-ounce) can no-salt-added light tuna, drained

1 large Hard-Boiled Egg (page 259), chopped

2 tablespoons finely chopped celery

1 tablespoon finely chopped red onion

1 tablespoon extra-virgin olive oil

1 tablespoon drained chopped capers

$1/4$ teaspoon grated lemon zest

1 teaspoon fresh lemon juice, or to taste

$1/8$ teaspoon salt

$1/8$ teaspoon freshly ground black pepper, or to taste

2 (6-inch) whole-wheat tortillas

$2/3$ cup broccoli or alfalfa sprouts (about $1^1/2$ ounces)
   or thinly shredded romaine lettuce

In a small bowl, place the tuna, hard-boiled egg, celery, onion, olive oil, capers, lemon zest and juice, salt, and pepper. Use a fork to gently loosen the tuna and combine it with the other ingredients. Taste and add more lemon juice or pepper, if desired.

Lay the tortillas on the work surface. Divide the tuna salad between them, arranging the salad in a straight line down the center of each. Spread the sprouts over each, dividing them evenly between the tortillas. Roll up each sandwich into a tight cylinder. Slice each in half and serve.

Calories: 419.5 kcal

Fat: 19.2 g

Protein: 33.0 g

Carbohydrates: 24.7 g

Sodium: 502.4 mg

ham and apple on grilled country bread SERVES 1

Olive oil spray, for the grill pan

2 slices crusty whole-wheat bread, such as boule or country loaf

$1^1/2$ teaspoons Dijon mustard

$^1/4$ teaspoon honey

$1^1/2$ ounces thinly sliced organic Black Forest or other smoked ham

$^1/2$ ounce reduced-fat Cheddar cheese, thinly sliced

$^1/4$ Granny Smith apple, cored and thinly sliced

Freshly ground black pepper to taste

Spray a grill pan with olive oil and heat over medium-high heat until hot but not smoking. Place the bread slices on the grill and grill until grill marks appear on both sides, about 2 minutes per side.

Meanwhile, in a small bowl, place the mustard and honey. Stir with a small spoon until well combined.

Place the grilled bread on a work surface and spread the mustard and honey mixture on both slices. On one slice of bread, place the ham, gently folding each slice in thirds to give the sandwich some height. Arrange the cheese slices on top and then the apple slices. Grind some black pepper on the apple. Place the other slice of grilled bread on top. Slice the sandwich in half. Serve.

Calories: 290.4 kcal

Fat: 6.1 g

Protein: 19.4 g

Carbohydrates: 39.8 g

Sodium: 860.8 mg

chicken salad with red grapes and toasted pecans

Who says you can't have chicken salad on a diet? You can if you use this alternative that does an end run around the fatty mayo. MAKES ABOUT 4 CUPS SALAD; ENOUGH FOR 6 SALAD SERVINGS OR 8 SANDWICHES

1 pound boneless, skinless chicken breast,
     poached (page 258) and cooled
1 cup halved red grapes
$1/3$ cup chopped pecans, toasted (page 96)
$1/3$ cup low-fat plain Greek yogurt
$1/4$ cup chopped celery
1 teaspoon honey
1 teaspoon cider vinegar
$1/4$ teaspoon salt
$1/8$ teaspoon ground black pepper

FOR 1 SANDWICH
2 slices whole-wheat sandwich bread
1 butterhead lettuce leaf

Use your fingers to shred the chicken into a large bowl. Add the grapes and pecans and toss gently to mix the ingredients. In a small bowl, stir together the yogurt, celery, honey, vinegar, salt, and pepper. Pour the dressing over the chicken and toss to coat. Store the salad in a tightly sealed container in the refrigerator for up to 3 days. Let stand at room temperature for about 15 minutes before serving.

To make a sandwich, toast the bread, if desired. Place $1/2$ cup chicken salad on 1 slice. Top with the lettuce leaf and the other slice of bread. Slice in half and serve.

Per $1/2$-cup serving of chicken salad:
Calories: 118.6 kcal
Fat: 5.1 g
Protein: 12.9 g
Carbohydrates: 5.6 g
Sodium: 93.8 mg

Per sandwich:
Calories: 209.4 kcal
Fat: 6.1 g
Protein: 16.9 g
Carbohydrates: 21.8 g
Sodium: 229.7 mg

poultry and meat main dishes

ALMOND-CRUSTED CHICKEN BREASTS

PAN-FRIED CHICKEN WITH FENNEL AND CARROTS

CHICKEN SATAY WITH ALMOND SAUCE

CHICKEN STIR-FRY WITH ASPARAGUS, RED PEPPER, AND SPINACH

ROASTED CHICKEN WITH WHOLE-WHEAT PASTA AND SPINACH PESTO

GRILLED LEMON CHICKEN

CURRIED CHICKEN WITH CILANTRO-LIME SAUCE

TANDOORI TURKEY KEBABS

ROASTED TURKEY BREAST WITH CRANBERRY-ORANGE SAUCE

GRILLED LAMB SKEWERS WITH PLUMS

MEDITERRANEAN LAMB BURGERS

PORK MEDALLIONS WITH POMEGRANATE SAUCE

ROASTED PORK STUFFED WITH ARTICHOKE, FETA, AND BLACK OLIVES

BEEF STIR-FRY WITH BROCCOLI AND SHIITAKE MUSHROOMS

GRILLED SKIRT STEAK WITH CHIMICHURRI SAUCE

almond-crusted chicken breasts

This nut topping comes together in minutes and keeps roasted chicken breasts tender and juicy in the oven. Serve with a green vegetable steamed in the microwave, (page 216), and your meal is ready in 20 minutes!

SERVES 4

$1/2$ cup unsalted almonds, toasted (page 96)
2 tablespoons extra-virgin olive oil
$3/4$ teaspoon grated lemon zest
1 tablespoon fresh lemon juice
$3/4$ teaspoon dried rosemary
1 garlic clove
$1/4$ teaspoon salt
4 (4- to 5-ounce) boneless, skinless chicken breast
    halves

Preheat the oven to 425°F.

In the work bowl of a food processor, place the almonds, olive oil, lemon zest and juice, rosemary, garlic, and salt. Process until coarsely chopped; the mixture will be a thick paste.

Arrange the chicken breast halves in a baking dish. Divide the almond paste and spread on the breasts; pat down to cover each breast completely.

Roast in the oven until cooked through and an instant-read thermometer reads 165° to 170°F, about 10 minutes. Loosely tent with foil and let stand for 5 to 10 minutes before serving.

Calories: 293.3 kcal
Fat: 17.4 g
Protein: 30.0 g
Carbohydrates: 4.3 g
Sodium: 194.2 mg

MASTERING POULTRY

Smart Selection

The recipes in this book call for 4- to 5-ounce boneless, skinless chicken breasts. If you can find only larger breasts, lay one breast at a time on a work surface. Holding a knife parallel to the work surface, cut straight through the length of the breast, creating a top portion that is uniformly thin. Use this top portion—where the skin was attached—for your recipe. Save the portion you removed for a stir-fry. Alternatively, simply cut them crosswise in half; for the recipes in this book, cook them a little longer if you cut them this way because they'll be thicker and require more time to cook all the way through.

When purchasing poultry, keep the following in mind:

- Make sure the texture of the poultry is plump and pliable.
- The skin should be opaque, not spotted.
- If purchasing frozen chicken, make sure it's frozen solid and has no freezer burn. Avoid chicken that has frozen liquid in the package, which indicates it has been frozen, defrosted, and refrozen.

Smart Storage

- Store poultry in the coldest place in your refrigerator. Under this condition it should keep for 2 to 3 days.
- Don't remove the chicken from its packaging until you are ready to prepare it. Make sure the package isn't leaking, or it can contaminate other things in your fridge.
- Poultry can also be stored in the freezer. Never defrost at room temperature. Instead, place the tightly wrapped frozen poultry in the refrigerator until defrosted. For faster defrosting, submerge the poultry—wrapped in leak-proof packaging—in a bowl of cold water. Change the water every 30 minutes. Or, you may use the "defrost" setting on your microwave; poultry defrosted this way must be cooked immediately, for some areas of the food may have begun to cook.

Smart Preparation

- When handling raw poultry, use separate cooking utensils and cutting boards.
- Broiling, roasting, grilling, and sautéing are all acceptable ways to cook poultry, but be sure not to burn or overcook it because free radicals that form can damage your health.
- You can cook it with the skin on so it remains moist, but—and you know this already—avoid eating the skin. It's full of saturated fats and unwanted extra calories.

pan-fried chicken with fennel and carrots

To release the flavor of fennel seed, crush it lightly in a mortar with a pestle or place it on a cutting board and add a few drops of water or the chicken broth. With a sharp knife, chop it several times to break up the seeds. SERVES 4

4 (4- to 5-ounce) boneless, skinless chicken breast halves
$1/2$ teaspoon ground cloves
Salt and ground black pepper
$1^1/2$ tablespoons virgin coconut oil
1 fennel bulb, trimmed, cored, and thinly sliced
2 large carrots, peeled and thinly sliced
1 red bell pepper, cored, seeded, and thinly sliced
1 teaspoon ground cumin
Grated zest and juice from 1 orange (about $1/2$ cup juice)
$1/2$ cup reduced-sodium chicken broth
1 teaspoon fennel seeds, lightly crushed
$1/4$ cup chopped parsley

Pat the chicken breasts dry with paper towels. In a small dish, place $1/4$ teaspoon of the cloves and $1/4$ teaspoon each salt and black pepper. Sprinkle both sides of the breasts with the clove mixture.

In a large skillet, heat 1 tablespoon of the oil over medium-high heat. Cook the chicken until lightly browned, 2 to 3 minutes per side. Transfer to a plate and set aside.

Reduce the heat to medium. Add the remaining $1/2$ tablespoon oil to the pan along with the fennel, carrots, and bell pepper. Cook, stirring occasionally, until crisp-tender and lightly browned, 5 to 7 minutes. Add the remaining $1/4$ teaspoon cloves, the cumin, a pinch of salt, and $1/4$ teaspoon pepper. Cook, stirring, until the spices are fragrant, about 30 seconds.

Add the orange zest and juice, the broth, and the crushed fennel seeds. Reduce the heat, cover, and simmer for 5 minutes. Remove the cover and add the reserved chicken to the skillet along with any accumulated juices. Simmer until the vegetables are soft and the chicken is opaque in the center, about 5 minutes. Divide the fennel mixture among four plates and place a chicken breast on top or alongside the fennel. Sprinkle parsley on top of the chicken and serve.

Calories: 206.7 kcal
Fat: 4.0 g
Protein: 28.7 g
Carbohydrates: 14.3 g
Sodium: 323.1 mg

Anti-Cancer Heart Healthy Boosts Metabolism Improves Mood Anti-Inflammatory

chicken satay with almond sauce

SERVES 4

1 pound boneless, skinless chicken breast
$^1/_2$ cup plus 1 teaspoon low-sodium tamari
Juice of 1 orange (about $^1/_2$ cup)
Juice of 1 lime (about $1^1/_2$ tablespoons)
3 garlic cloves, chopped
$^1/_4$ cup rice wine vinegar
2 tablespoons natural almond butter
1 tablespoon honey
1 tablespoon minced fresh ginger
$^1/_4$ teaspoon toasted sesame oil
Olive oil spray, for the grill

WHAT'S IN THERE?!: IRRADIATED MEAT

So gross. I mean . . . really? Here's what happens: conventionally raised animals are kept in horrifying conditions, where they basically sit in their own excrement until the day they are slaughtered. The bacteria from their feces are on and in the meat—think *E. coli* and the like—so, to be safe, meat is irradiated to prolong its shelf life and reduce the risk of food poisoning.

You can tell if your meat has been so treated by looking for the words "irradiated" or "pasteurized" on the packaging. Currently more than 3,000 supermarkets in America, as well as our nation's school-lunch program, carry irradiated meat. This is a relatively new practice, so we don't know how serious the health ramifications are for humans yet. With that said, the European Union is concerned about the chemicals that irradiation creates in the meat and is pursuing further studies. I don't know about you, but the "maybe" game is just not something I want to play where my health is concerned.

What's the best way to avoid this? Going organic, of course. Or, if organic is not affordable, opt for fish instead of beef or chicken.

Slice the chicken breast into thin strips 3 to 4 inches long; this is easier to do if the chicken is placed in the freezer for 20 minutes before slicing. You should have about 40 slices (count out and set aside roughly half as many wooden skewers as you have slices of chicken). In a medium bowl, mix the $1/2$ cup tamari, the orange juice, lime juice, and 2 of the garlic cloves. Add the chicken slices. Cover the bowl and refrigerate for at least 1 hour and up to overnight.

Before you are ready to grill the chicken, soak the wooden skewers in water for at least 20 minutes.

Meanwhile, in a blender or the work bowl of a food processor, place the vinegar, almond butter, honey, ginger, sesame oil, 1 teaspoon tamari, and remaining garlic clove. Blend or process until smooth. Set aside until ready to serve.

If using a gas or charcoal grill, spray the grill with olive oil and prepare a medium-hot grill. If using a grill pan, spray it with olive oil and heat over medium-high heat.

Pat the chicken slices dry, and thread 2 slices onto each skewer. Grill for 2 to 3 minutes per side. Arrange the hot skewers on a platter and either drizzle the sauce over or serve the sauce in a bowl alongside the skewers.

Calories: 203.5 kcal

Fat: 5.5 g

Protein: 29.0 g

Carbohydrates: 9.1 g

Sodium: 596.8 mg

chicken stir-fry with asparagus, red pepper, and spinach SERVES 4

2 tablespoons rice wine vinegar

1 tablespoon plus 2 teaspoons toasted sesame oil

1 tablespoon fresh lime juice

1^1/$_2$ teaspoons honey

^{1}/$_2$ teaspoon minced red or green fresh chiles

1 pound boneless, skinless chicken breast, cut into
    bite-size pieces

1 tablespoon low-sodium tamari

1^1/$_2$ tablespoons virgin coconut oil

2 garlic cloves, minced

1 tablespoon finely grated fresh ginger

^{1}/$_2$ red onion, thinly sliced

2 large bell peppers, cored, seeded, and thinly sliced
    into 1-inch pieces

8 ounces asparagus, sliced lengthwise if thick, cut into
    1-inch pieces

^{2}/$_3$ cup low-sodium chicken broth

5 cups packed spinach, coarsely chopped

Brown Rice (page 261)

2 tablespoons sesame seeds, toasted (page 96)

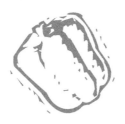

In a small bowl, whisk together 1 tablespoon of the vinegar, 1 tablespoon of the sesame oil, the lime juice, 1/2 teaspoon of the honey, and the chiles. Add the chicken, cover, and refrigerate, preferably for at least 30 minutes and up to 4 hours.

In a small bowl, whisk together the tamari with the remaining 1 tablespoon vinegar, the remaining 2 teaspoons sesame oil, and the remaining 1 teaspoon honey to make the stir-fry sauce. Set aside.

When ready to stir-fry, drain the marinated chicken and discard the marinade.

Heat a wok or large skillet (not nonstick) over high heat for about 20 seconds. When it is hot, add the coconut oil. As soon as the oil is melted, add the garlic and ginger and cook, stirring, until fragrant, about 10 seconds. Add the onion and cook, stirring, until slightly softened, 30 seconds to 1 minute. Add the chicken and cook, stirring, for 30 seconds. Add the bell peppers and asparagus and cook, stirring, until well coated in oil and beginning to soften, about 1 minute. Add the chicken broth, cover the pan, and cook for 3 to 4 minutes, until the vegetables are softened but still brightly colored. Add the spinach and the stir-fry sauce, and toss well. Remove from the heat.

Divide the rice among four plates and top with the chicken stir-fry. Sprinkle the sesame seeds over each plate and serve.

Calories: 388.4 kcal

Fat: 12.4 g

Protein: 33.7 g

Carbohydrates: 35.6 g

Sodium: 274.9 mg

*Nutritional analysis does not include the rice (see page 261).

roasted chicken with whole-wheat pasta and spinach pesto

This method for roasting a boneless chicken breast can be used for preparing chicken to add to any salad or small side dish to make it a complete meal. Here, it is seasoned with cinnamon, whose warm flavor enhances the spinach pesto. But for another dish, top the chicken with 1 teaspoon dried rosemary or your favorite dried herb.

SERVES 6

1 whole boneless, skinless chicken breast
   (3/4 to 1 pound)
$^1/_4$ cup plus 1 teaspoon extra-virgin olive oil
$^1/_4$ teaspoon ground cinnamon
Salt and ground black pepper
2 bunches flat-leaf spinach ($1^1/_2$ pounds total),
   trimmed
1 cup packed fresh parsley leaves
10 ounces whole-wheat short tubular pasta,
   such as rigatoni
$^1/_3$ cup ($1^1/_4$ ounces) walnuts, toasted (page 96)
$^1/_4$ cup ($3/_4$ ounce) grated Parmesan cheese
2 garlic cloves
2 teaspoons tomato paste
1 teaspoon grated lemon zest
1 tablespoon fresh lemon juice
1 pint cherry tomatoes, halved

Preheat the oven to 425°F. Bring a large pot of water to a boil. Prepare a large bowl of ice water.

Place the chicken breast in a small baking dish. Drizzle with 1 teaspoon of the olive oil. In a small dish, combine $1/8$ teaspoon of the cinnamon with a pinch of salt and pepper. Sprinkle the cinnamon mixture over the chicken. Bake, uncovered, until an instant-read thermometer reads 165° to 170°F, 15 to 20 minutes. Set aside.

Meanwhile, prepare the pesto. Stir the spinach and parsley into the boiling water, in batches if necessary. Cook until wilted and bright green, about 30 seconds. Immediately transfer the greens to the ice bath to stop the cooking. Repeat until all of the spinach and the parsley are wilted. When completely cool, drain the greens well and transfer them to a clean kitchen towel. Squeeze the towel to extract as much liquid as possible. Set aside.

Return the water to a boil. Cook the pasta in the boiling water until al dente, 12 to 15 minutes or according to package instructions. Reserve $1/2$ cup pasta cooking water; then drain the pasta and return it to the pot.

Meanwhile, place the spinach and parsley in a food processor. Add the walnuts, Parmesan cheese, garlic, tomato paste, lemon zest and juice, and remaining $1/8$ teaspoon cinnamon. Process to a coarse paste. With the motor running, pour in the remaining $1/4$ cup olive oil and $1/4$ cup tap water; process until smooth and creamy, 1 to 2 minutes. Season with $1/4$ teaspoon salt and $1/4$ teaspoon pepper.

Add the tomatoes and pesto to the pasta; toss, adding the reserved pasta water to coat the pasta, if necessary. Divide the chicken breast into 2 halves and slice each one thinly. Divide the pasta among six plates and top with the chicken. Serve.

Calories: 450.3 kcal

Fat: 18.3 g

Protein: 22.7 g

Carbohydrates: 51.7 g

Sodium: 430.8 mg

grilled lemon chicken This simple method yields tangy-sweet and super-moist chicken, perfect for serving with Russet Potato Salad with Arugula and Lemon (page 212) or green vegetables steamed in the microwave (page 216). SERVES 6

1 teaspoon lemon zest
Juice of 1 lemon
$1/4$ cup chopped fresh basil or oregano
1 tablespoon honey
1 tablespoon Dijon mustard
2 garlic cloves, minced
$1/2$ teaspoon salt
$1/4$ teaspoon black pepper
$1/4$ cup extra-virgin olive oil
6 (4- to 5-ounce) boneless, skinless chicken breast
    halves
$1/4$ cup pitted kalamata olives, halved
Olive oil spray, for the grill

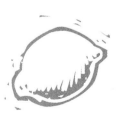

To prepare the dressing, whisk together the lemon zest and juice, the basil, honey, mustard, garlic, and salt and pepper. Whisking constantly, add the olive oil in a slow stream. Set aside.

Place the chicken on a cutting board and lay a sheet of wax paper over it. Using the flat side of a meat mallet, pound the chicken slightly so it is an even thickness. Place the chicken in a shallow baking dish just large enough to hold it. Pour half of the dressing (about 1/3 cup) over the chicken and turn the breasts once or twice to coat. Cover the dish and refrigerate for at least 2 hours if possible, and up to 8 hours, turning at least once.

Stir the olives into the remaining dressing, and set aside until ready to serve.

If using a gas or charcoal grill, spray the grill with olive oil and prepare a medium-hot grill. If using a grill pan, spray it with olive oil and heat over medium-high heat.

Discard the marinade and grill the chicken until it is opaque in the center, 5 to 6 minutes per side.

Place the chicken on a platter and drizzle with the dressing. Serve.

Calories: 227.3 kcal
Fat: 11.1 g
Protein: 26.6 g
Carbohydrates: 3.9 g
Sodium: 395.4 mg

curried chicken with cilantro-lime sauce
This is especially delicious served with Coconut-Ginger Yellow Rice (page 208). Begin the preparation of the rice, or any other long-cooking grain dish, before you cook the chicken so it's all ready to serve at the same time. SERVES 4

FOR THE CURRY CHICKEN
1 tablespoon virgin coconut oil
1 teaspoon red curry paste
4 (4- to 5-ounce) boneless, skinless chicken breast
    halves
$1/2$ cup low-sodium chicken broth
1 teaspoon honey

FOR THE CILANTRO-LIME SAUCE
2 packed cups cilantro leaves
2 tablespoons fresh lime juice
1 tablespoon olive oil
1 teaspoon honey
1 to 2 teaspoons finely chopped green chile (optional)
1 garlic clove, chopped
$1/2$ teaspoon chopped fresh ginger
$1/2$ teaspoon garam masala
$1/4$ teaspoon salt

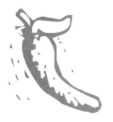

To prepare the chicken, in a large skillet over medium-low heat, add the oil and curry paste and heat, stirring, until combined. Add the chicken and cook for 2 minutes. Turn and cook for 1 minute. In a separate bowl, combine the chicken broth and the honey and stir to blend. Pour over the chicken and bring to a boil. Reduce the heat, cover, and simmer very gently until the chicken is cooked, about 15 minutes.

While the chicken is cooking, prepare the Cilantro-Lime Sauce. In a blender, place the cilantro, lime juice, olive oil, honey, and chile, if using; add the garlic, ginger, garam masala, salt, and 3 tablespoons water. Puree until smooth, adding another tablespoon of water, if necessary. Set aside.

When the chicken is cooked, transfer it to a plate and gently tent with aluminum foil to keep warm. Simmer the liquid in the pan until reduced and thickened. Return the chicken to the pan and flip each breast once or twice to coat with sauce. Spoon the remaining Cilantro-Lime Sauce over the chicken and serve.

For the chicken with the sauce:
Calories: 206.0 kcal
Fat: 8.5 g
Protein: 26.8 g
Carbohydrates: 4.7 g
Sodium: 273.3 mg

For the Cilantro-Lime Sauce alone:
Calories: 53.7 kcal
Fat: 3.6 g
Protein: 0.3 g
Carbohydrates: 5.7 g
Sodium: 124.4 mg

HEALTH BENEFITS:

**Anti-Cancer Heart Healthy Boosts Immunity Boosts Metabolism Improves Mood
Anti-Inflammatory Improves Digestion Miscellaneous**

tandoori turkey kebabs SERVES 4

$1/2$ cup nonfat plain yogurt
2 teaspoons fresh lime juice
1 teaspoon chopped fresh ginger
1 garlic clove, chopped
$1/2$ teaspoon ground cumin
$1/2$ teaspoon turmeric
$1/4$ teaspoon ground black pepper
$1/8$ teaspoon salt
1 pound boneless, skinless turkey breast, cut into
    $1^1/2$-inch pieces
Olive oil spray, for the grill
Cilantro-Lime Sauce (page 124), for serving

In a medium bowl, combine the yogurt, lime juice, ginger, garlic, cumin, turmeric, pepper, and salt. Add the turkey and marinate for at least 10 minutes and up to overnight.

Place 8 wooden skewers in a pan of water and let soak for at least 20 minutes.

If using a gas or charcoal grill, spray the grill with olive oil and prepare a medium-hot grill. If using a grill pan, spray it with olive oil and heat over medium-high heat.

Thread the turkey onto the skewers. Grill, turning occasionally, until cooked through, 10 to 12 minutes. Serve with the Cilantro-Lime Sauce.

Calories: 182.3 kcal
Fat: 4.1 g
Protein: 29.0 g
Carbohydrates: 7.4 g
Sodium: 263.2 mg
*Nutritional analysis includes the
Cilantro-Lime Sauce.

MASTER GRILLING

For safe grilling and good barbecue, propane gas grills are the way to go. They emit less carbon into the atmosphere than charcoal (producing 5.6 pounds of carbon an hour compared to 11 pounds from charcoal). Still, if you prefer charcoal because of the taste, be sure to go natural so the charcoal won't give off harmful chemicals. Some good options are recycled wood, coconut shells, and corncob briquettes. In addition, make sure you use leaner cuts of meat that won't create fat-drip flare-ups. These flare-ups deposit known carcinogens, called heterocyclic amines (HCAs) or polycyclic aromatic hydrocarbons (PAHs), onto the meat. HCAs and PAHs are also found in well-done meat, so keep these harmful toxins at bay by cooking your meat on the rarer side.

For most people, determining how long to grill meat can be a bit confusing. Don't sweat it—just follow this chart. Try to turn your meat only once, in the middle of the total cooking time, to allow the meat to brown just right.

Meat	Grill Time
Burgers	5 to 8 minutes each side (10 to 16 minutes total)
Chicken breast	4 to 6 minutes each side (8 to 12 minutes total)
Fish fillet ($1/2$-inch-thick)	2 to 3 minutes each side (4 to 6 minutes total)
Fish steak (1-inch-thick)	4 to 6 minutes each side (8 to 12 minutes total)
Lamb chops	6 to 8 minutes each side (12 to 16 minutes total)
Pork chops	6 to 8 minutes each side (12 to 16 minutes total)
Pork tenderloin	6 to 9 minutes each side (12 to 18 minutes total; keep turning the meat)
Shrimp	3 to 4 minutes each side (6 to 8 minutes total)
Grass-fed beef steak	4 to 6 minutes each side (8 to 12 minutes total)

roasted turkey breast with cranberry-orange sauce

This elegant dish is perfect for entertaining during the holidays and is fabulous served with Smashed Sweet Potatoes with Coconut Milk (page 223)—just be sure to double that recipe if you're serving 8 with this one! You may be able to find skinless, boneless, butterflied turkey breast sold as "turkey London broil." In this case, you can skip the first step below, in which the turkey is butterflied. If you can find only boneless turkey breast with the skin, simply remove and discard the skin before butterflying the breast. SERVES 8

1 boneless, skinless turkey breast (about 2^1/2 pounds)
2 teaspoons chopped parsley
2 teaspoons chopped fresh rosemary, plus sprigs for garnish
2 teaspoons chopped fresh sage, plus sprigs for garnish
1 teaspoon chopped fresh thyme leaves
^{1}/2 teaspoon salt
^{1}/4 teaspoon freshly ground black pepper
1 tablespoon olive oil
Up to ^{1}/2 cup low-sodium chicken broth
^{1}/2 cup fresh orange juice (from 1 to 2 oranges)
^{1}/2 cup fresh or frozen cranberries
2 teaspoons honey

Position a rack in the center of the oven. Preheat oven to 350°F.

Place the turkey breast on a work surface skin side down. Holding a sharp knife parallel to the work surface, start at the middle of the breast and cut a deep incision into the thickest part of the meat, cutting toward the outer edge of the breast; be very careful not to cut all the way through. Open this flap like a book. Repeat on the other side. Open this flap out to the other side. Cover the turkey with a sheet of wax paper. Using the flat side of a meat mallet, pound the breast gently to flatten it evenly.

In a small bowl, combine the parsley, rosemary, sage, and thyme. Sprinkle the herbs over the cut surface of the roast. Starting at a short end, roll the breast into a thick cylinder. Tie crosswise in three or four places with kitchen string. Season the outside of the roast with the salt and pepper.

In a Dutch oven or flameproof casserole slightly larger than the turkey breast, heat the olive oil over medium-high heat. Add the breast and cook, turning occasionally, until browned on all sides, about 10 minutes. Cover tightly and bake until an instant-read thermometer inserted in the center of the breast reads 160° to 165°F, about 30 minutes. Transfer the turkey breast to a carving board and loosely tent with aluminum foil to keep warm.

Pour the cooking juices out of the pot into a 1-cup glass measure. Let stand for a few minutes, and then skim off the fat that rises to the surface using a spoon or paper towels. Add enough chicken broth to the cooking juices to make 1/2 cup. Return the liquid to the pot and add the orange juice, cranberries, and honey. Bring to a boil over high heat. Boil until the cranberries have popped and the sauce is slightly thickened and has reduced to about 2/3 cup, about 5 minutes. Stir in any juices from the turkey.

Thinly slice the turkey and divide among eight plates. Pour the sauce over each plate and serve.

Calories: 190.1 kcal
Fat: 1.1 g
Protein: 34.5 g
Carbohydrates: 8.7 g
Sodium: 187.4 mg

grilled lamb skewers with plums

The flavors of warm spices and the deep chocolate undertones of this dish beautifully complement earthy lamb. I know that not everyone is a fan of lamb, so feel free to substitute grass-fed beef if you prefer it. Serve with mixed greens tossed with Fruit Vinaigrette (page 263), made with pitted plums. SERVES 4

1 tablespoon natural (not Dutch-processed) unsweetened cocoa powder

1 tablespoon plus $1/4$ teaspoon ground cinnamon

1 tablespoon dried thyme

$1/4$ teaspoon ground cloves

$1/2$ teaspoon salt

$1/2$ teaspoon ground black pepper

1 pound boneless lamb top round, cut into $1^{1}/2$-inch cubes

3 teaspoons olive oil

4 ripe plums, pitted and cut into 4 wedges

Olive oil spray, for the grill

2 teaspoons sherry vinegar, for serving (optional)

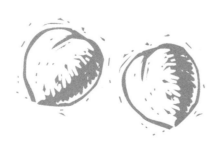

Place 12 wooden skewers in water and let soak for at least 20 minutes.

Meanwhile, in a small bowl, combine the cocoa, 1 tablespoon of the cinnamon, the thyme, cloves, and salt and pepper.

Pat the lamb cubes dry, and then place them in a bowl, pouring 2 teaspoons of the olive oil over the lamb. Toss to coat the meat with oil. Roll each cube in the spice mix and turn until all sides are coated. Thread the lamb cubes onto 8 of the skewers, dividing equally.

Thread 4 plum wedges on each of the remaining 4 skewers. Brush the plums with the remaining 1 teaspoon olive oil and sprinkle some of the remaining ¼ teaspoon ground cinnamon over each plum.

If using a gas or charcoal grill, spray the grill with olive oil and prepare a medium-hot grill. If using a grill pan, spray it with olive oil and heat over medium-high heat.

Grill the lamb, turning occasionally, until cooked to the desired doneness, 6 to 7 minutes for medium-rare. Grill the plums, turning occasionally, until they are softened but not mushy and have marks in places, 5 to 10 minutes. Transfer the skewers to a platter. If desired, drizzle with the sherry vinegar while hot. Serve.

Calories: 287.1 kcal
Fat: 12.3 g
Protein: 32.8 g
Carbohydrates: 10.8 g
Sodium: 328.1 mg

mediterranean lamb burgers These

flavorful burgers are delicious served with Creamy

Cucumber and Yogurt Salad (page 214). SERVES 4

$^1/_4$ cup ($1^1/_4$ ounces) sunflower seeds
$^1/_4$ cup ($^3/_4$ ounce) rolled oats (not instant)
1 teaspoon fresh oregano leaves, or $^1/_4$ teaspoon dried
1 teaspoon fresh mint leaves, or $^1/_4$ teaspoon dried
Grated zest from 1 lemon
1 pound ground lamb
1 tablespoon tahini
1 garlic clove, minced
$^1/_4$ teaspoon salt
$^1/_2$ teaspoon ground black pepper

In the work bowl of a food processor, place the sunflower seeds, rolled oats, oregano, mint, and lemon zest. Process until ground but not mushy or pureed.

Place the lamb in a large mixing bowl and add the sunflower seed mixture along with the tahini, garlic, salt, and pepper. Use your hands to gently combine. Form the mixture into four $3^1/_2$-inch patties and place on a plate.

Heat a large cast-iron or other heavy-bottomed (not nonstick) skillet over medium heat. When the skillet is hot, add the burgers and cook for 5 to 6 minutes, then turn them with a spatula. Cook for another 5 to 6 minutes. Serve hot.

Calories: 315.1 kcal
Fat: 21.8 g
Protein: 22.7 g
Carbohydrates: 7.4 g
Sodium: 185.9 mg

MASTERING MEAT

Smart Selection: Beef, Lamb, Venison

- Buy the freshest meat possible. Check the sell-by date and pick the package of meat with the latest expiration.
- Make sure the meat is red or purplish in color and not gray or brown, which is an indication that the meat is spoiled or spoiling.
- Select the meat with the least amount of fat running through it. The fat that runs through the meat should be white, not yellow. Yellow fat indicates the animal was sick or old.

Smart Selection: Pork

- Select pork that's pinkish-white to pink in color (loin meat is whiter than shoulder meat) and is firm to the touch.

Smart Storage

- Meat can be stored in the freezer or in the refrigerator.
- Place the meat in a plastic airtight bag to prevent spoiling and leakage. In general I don't believe in using plastic of any kind, since whatever wrap you put around your food will be on this planet centuries from now, but for safety's sake sometimes it's necessary; please use it judiciously and look for bisphenol-A (BPA)- and polyvinyl chloride (PVC)–free brands.

Smart Preparation

- Use a separate cutting board and cooking utensils when preparing meat to protect yourself and your family against *E. coli* contamination.
- Meat can be thawed in the fridge or at room temperature. To thaw at room temperature, put the meat in a watertight plastic bag and place it in a bowl of cold water. Change the water every 30 minutes.
- Don't overcook or burn meat, as free radicals can form that are potentially harmful to your health. See page 160 for USDA-recommended internal temperatures for cooked meat.

pork medallions with pomegranate sauce

Pomegranate is great for disrupting the damaging effects of "bad" LDL cholesterol—at least that's what current research suggests—which helps keep your arteries clear and your heart healthy. The seeds themselves are actually covered with sweet, juicy flesh; you can eat the whole thing. The season for pomegranates is short, but you can enjoy the seeds longer with careful storage. Kept in a tightly sealed container, they can be refrigerated for up to 3 days or frozen for up to 6 months. Frozen seeds should be used in cooked recipes, such as this one.

SERVES 4

1 pomegranate
1 pound boneless pork tenderloin, sliced into
    $1/2$-inch-thick medallions
$1/4$ teaspoon salt
$1/4$ teaspoon pepper
3 teaspoons olive oil
$1/2$ cup finely chopped red onion
1 cup plain pomegranate juice
$1/4$ cup reduced-sodium chicken broth
1 tablespoon honey
1 tablespoon balsamic vinegar
3 sprigs fresh thyme

Cut the pomegranate in half through the stem. Fill a large bowl with water. Holding the pomegranate under the water, remove the seeds with your hands. Drain the seeds well. Set aside $1/3$ cup. Reserve the rest for another use.

Season the medallions with the salt and pepper.

Heat 2 teaspoons of the olive oil in a skillet over medium-high heat and cook the pork until light pink in the center, 2 or 3 minutes per side. Transfer to a plate and tent loosely with foil to keep warm.

Turn the heat to medium and add the remaining 1 teaspoon oil to the skillet. Add the onion and cook, stirring, until softened, about 3 minutes. Stir in the pomegranate juice, chicken broth, honey, vinegar, and thyme. Simmer until the sauce is reduced to about $1/2$ cup, 5 to 8 minutes.

Divide the medallions evenly among four plates and pour the sauce over each serving. Sprinkle each serving with pomegranate seeds and serve.

Calories: 243.5 kcal

Fat: 7.5 g

Protein: 24.8 g

Carbohydrates: 18.6 g

Sodium: 191.3 mg

roasted pork stuffed with artichoke, feta, and black olives

SERVES 4

3 ounces frozen artichoke hearts, thawed

3 tablespoons crumbled reduced-fat feta cheese (3/4 ounce)

3 tablespoons coarsely chopped kalamata olives

1 teaspoon finely chopped fresh oregano leaves

3/4 teaspoon lemon zest

3/4 teaspoon fresh lemon juice

1/4 teaspoon salt

1/2 teaspoon ground black pepper

1 pound boneless pork tenderloin

1 teaspoon olive oil

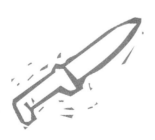

Preheat the oven to 450°F.

Press the artichokes between towels to remove any excess moisture. In the work bowl of a food processor, place the artichokes, feta, olives, oregano, lemon zest and juice, 1/8 teaspoon of the salt, and 1/4 teaspoon of the pepper. Pulse until the artichokes and olives are finely chopped, scraping the side of the bowl occasionally.

Pat the meat dry with paper towels and place it on a cutting board. Holding a sharp knife parallel to the cutting board, make a cut down the center of one long side of the tenderloin, cutting to, but not through, the opposite side. Open the meat like a book, so it lies flat. Lay a sheet of wax paper over the meat. Using the flat side of a meat mallet, pound the pork to an even 1/2-inch thickness.

Spread the artichoke mixture evenly on half of the pork to within 1/4 inch of the edges. Fold the tenderloin in half to form its original shape. Tie closed with butcher's string at 1 1/2-inch intervals. Brush the pork with the olive oil and sprinkle with the remaining salt and pepper.

Place the pork, seam side up, on a rack in a shallow baking dish. Roast in the oven until an instant-read thermometer inserted in the thickest part of the roast reads 155° to 160°F, 15 to 20 minutes. Transfer the tenderloin to a clean cutting board and loosely tent with foil; let stand for 5 to 10 minutes.

To serve, remove the string and cut the pork into 1/2- to 3/4-inch slices.

Calories: 190.3 kcal
Fat: 8.5 g
Protein: 24.4 g
Carbohydrates: 3.2 g
Sodium: 417.6 mg

Anti-Cancer Heart Healthy Boosts Immunity Boosts Metabolism Improves Digestion Strong Bones

beef stir-fry with broccoli and shiitake mushrooms SERVES 4

4 cups broccoli florets (about 3/4 pound)
1 pound flank or boneless sirloin steak
Juice of 1 orange
Juice of 1 lime
1 teaspoon low-sodium tamari
1 teaspoon toasted sesame oil
1 tablespoon virgin coconut oil
1/2 cup thinly sliced scallions (green and white parts)
1 tablespoon minced garlic
1 tablespoon minced fresh ginger
1/4 teaspoon crushed red pepper flakes
4 ounces shiitake mushrooms, stemmed and sliced
1/4 cup (1 ounce) chopped Brazil nuts, toasted
    (page 96)
Brown Rice (page 261)

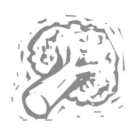

Prepare a bowl of ice water. Place the broccoli in a microwave-safe bowl. Cover and microwave on high power until bright green and slightly softened but still crunchy, 2 to 3 minutes. Drain the broccoli and immediately transfer to the ice water to stop the cooking. Drain well and set aside.

Slice the beef into thin strips about 3 inches long; this is easier to do if the meat is placed in the freezer for about 20 minutes before slicing.

In a small bowl, combine the orange and lime juices, tamari, and sesame oil. Set aside.

Heat a large skillet or wok (not nonstick) over high heat for 20 seconds. Add the coconut oil. When the oil is melted, add the scallions and cook, stirring, until softened, about 30 seconds. Then add the garlic, ginger, and red pepper flakes and cook, stirring, until fragrant and just lightly browned, about 30 seconds. Add the beef and cook until no longer pink, about 2 minutes. Stir in the reserved broccoli and cook for about 1 minute. Next, add the mushrooms and continue to stir while cooking for 1 to 2 minutes.

Stir in the orange juice mixture and combine. Remove the skillet from the heat and mix in the nuts. Divide the cooked rice among four plates. Divide the beef stir-fry among the plates and serve.

Calories: 399.7 kcal
Fat: 16.7 g
Protein: 31.5 g
Carbohydrates: 32.7 g
Sodium: 141.2 mg
*Nutritional analysis does not include the rice (see page 261).

grilled skirt steak with chimichurri sauce SERVES 4

$1/4$ cup chopped red onion
3 garlic cloves
$1/2$ teaspoon crushed red pepper flakes
$1/2$ cup packed flat-leaf parsley leaves
2 tablespoons packed fresh oregano leaves
$1/4$ cup extra-virgin olive oil
2 tablespoons red wine vinegar
$1/4$ teaspoon salt
$1/2$ teaspoon black pepper
1 pound skirt steak
Olive oil spray, for the grill

In the work bowl of a food processor, place the onion, garlic, and red pepper flakes. Pulse until finely chopped. Add the parsley and oregano leaves, and pulse until the herbs are coarsely chopped. Add the olive oil, vinegar, and salt and pepper.

Place the skirt steak in a shallow pan and pour $1/3$ cup of the chimichurri sauce over it. Turn to coat well. Cover and refrigerate, preferably for at least 4 hours and up to overnight. Cover and refrigerate the remaining sauce.

If using a gas or charcoal grill, spray the grill with olive oil and prepare a medium-hot grill. If using a grill pan, spray it with olive oil and heat over medium-high heat.

Grill the steak for 4 to 5 minutes per side for medium-rare. Let stand on a cutting board for 5 to 10 minutes. Thinly slice the steak and divide among four plates. Top each serving with 1 generous teaspoon of chimichurri sauce and serve.

Calories: 339.2 kcal
Fat: 25.1 g
Protein: 24.3 g
Carbohydrates: 2.8 g
Sodium: 193.2 mg

fish and shellfish main dishes

THAI GREEN CURRY BARRAMUNDI

POLLOCK IN PARCHMENT

BROILED TILAPIA WITH FRESH HERBS, MUSHROOMS, AND TOMATOES

GRILLED HALIBUT WITH FRESH BERRY AND GINGER SALSA

ROASTED SALMON WITH PEPITA AND CUMIN SEED CRUST

POACHED SALMON WITH GREEN GODDESS YOGURT

SPICY MAHI-MAHI AND MANGO TACOS

PECAN-CRUSTED CATFISH WITH CRANBERRY-MAPLE COMPOTE

ALMOND-ORANGE RAINBOW TROUT WITH CHIPOTLE YOGURT SAUCE

BROILED MACKEREL WITH LEMON-CAPER VINAIGRETTE

GRILLED SARDINES WITH LEMON AND BASIL

LINGUINE WITH ANCHOVIES, GARLIC, AND PARSLEY

COCONUT-CURRY STEAMED MUSSELS

MUSSELS WITH LINGUINE

BAY SCALLOPS WITH TOASTED SESAME SEEDS

CHILI-LIME SHRIMP SKEWERS WITH PINEAPPLE-MINT SALSA

GINGER SHRIMP ROLLS WITH GREEN PAPAYA SLAW

CALAMARI WITH SALSA VERDE AND ARUGULA

thai green curry barramundi

SERVES 4

1 tablespoon virgin coconut oil
1 cup thinly sliced red onion
1 cup thinly sliced carrots
1 tablespoon green curry paste, or to taste
$^2/_3$ cup coconut milk
4 (4-ounce) barramundi or halibut fillets, rinsed and
   patted dry
$^1/_4$ cup chopped cilantro leaves
Lime wedges, for serving

In a large skillet, heat the oil over medium heat. Add the onion and carrots and cook, stirring occasionally, until the onion is softened, about 4 minutes.

Stir in the green curry paste, and cook for 1 minute. Stir in the coconut milk and bring to a simmer.

Lay the fillets skin side down in the pan, moving the vegetables to the side to make room as you add each fillet. Pile the vegetables on top of the fillets, cover the pan, and simmer for 10 minutes, until the fish is opaque and flakes easily with a fork.

Place a fillet on each of four plates and spoon the vegetables and sauce over the fish. Sprinkle the cilantro over each serving and garnish with lime wedges. Serve.

Calories: 245.6 kcal
Fat: 13.6 g
Protein: 22.8 g
Carbohydrates: 9.1 g
Sodium: 114.8 mg

MASTERING FISH AND SHELLFISH: SMART SELECTION

Fish

- Make sure the fish smells fresh. If it has a strong, fishy smell, put it back.
- The flesh of the fish should have no discoloration.
- When you gently push the meat of the fish, it should bounce back and not remain dented.
- The gills of whole fish should be bright red.
- To avoid contamination from bacteria and food poisoning, do not purchase cooked seafood if it's in the same case as raw seafood.
- If you're concerned about the sustainability of seafood, with the information changing almost daily, the best way to stay abreast is to check the regional and national guidelines put out by Monterey Bay Aquarium's Seafood Watch program (www.sea foodwatch.org) or visit the World's Healthiest Foods Web site, www.whfoods.org.

Mollusks

- Mollusks (clams, oysters, mussels, or scallops) in the shell should always be alive when you buy them. When a mollusk is alive, the shells will be tightly closed or will close when tapped lightly or placed on ice. One way to test for freshness is to hold the shell between your thumb and forefinger and press as though sliding the two parts of the shell across each other. If the shells move, the shellfish is not fresh. Throw away any that do not close tightly.
- Buy farmed, not wild, mollusks. Clams, oysters, scallops, and mussels are the ideal farmed seafood. In the wild, they may be harvested using hydraulic dredges, which rip up the ocean floor; farming, on the other hand, involves either raising the mollusks on beaches and hand-raking to harvest (which has very little impact on the beach itself) or growing them on strings that hang from floating platforms or in metal-mesh sacks laid on floating racks. Neither method does any environmental damage.

Shellfish

- Shellfish (lobster, shrimp, crab) should have firm bodies attached to their shells.
- Make sure the flesh is not discolored with black spots. This is a sign of decay.
- The shell should not appear yellow or deteriorated. This is also a sign of decay.
- Shrimp is best when purchased frozen. Lobster and crab are best fresh.
- The shellfish should have a mild smell. If it smells strongly of seawater, do not eat it.

This Fish Is a Keeper

Here are my suggestions for the best and worst choices for fish, mollusks, and shellfish:

Go with These	Stay Away from These
Abalone	Atlantic cod
Alaska wild salmon (fresh, frozen, or canned)	Atlantic flounder/sole
	Atlantic halibut
Anchovies	Blue and king crab
Atlantic char	Bluefin tuna
Atlantic herring	Bluefish
Atlantic mackerel	Chilean sea bass
Barramundi (U.S. farm raised, not imported)	Croaker
	Eel
Black sea bass	Grouper
Clams (steamers)	King mackerel
Halibut	Lingcod
Mahi-mahi	Marlin
Oysters and mussels (farm raised)	Orange roughy
Pacific cod	Pacific roughy
Pacific halibut	Shad
Pollock	Shark
Rainbow trout (farm raised)	Summer and winter flounder
Red snapper	Swordfish
Rockfish	Wahoo
Sablefish	White sea bass
Sardines	Wild striped bass
Shrimp (farm raised)	Wild sturgeon
Stone, kona, and dungeness crab	
Tilapia (farm raised)	
Tilefish	
Tuna (canned light or albacore from U.S. and Canada)	

pollock in parchment

Make sure everyone is ready to eat when these come out of the oven. Part of the fun of this method is placing a packet in front of each diner and allowing him or her to experience firsthand the unbelievable aromas that pour out of the packets when they're ripped open. This works great for any delicate white fish, including cod and tilapia.

SERVES 4

4 (4-ounce) fillets pollock, cod, tilapia, or other white fish, rinsed and patted dry
2 teaspoons extra-virgin olive oil
$1/2$ teaspoon salt
$1/4$ teaspoon pepper
4 ounces shiitake mushrooms, stems trimmed, caps thinly sliced
2 to 3 strips lemon zest, removed with a vegetable peeler and thinly sliced lengthwise
4 tablespoons thinly shredded fresh basil leaves
$1/2$ cup thinly sliced red onion

Preheat the oven to 425°F. Prepare four 15-inch squares of parchment paper. Have ready 2 baking sheets.

Fold the parchment squares in half so they form rectangles. Close to the fold on one half of each sheet of parchment, place a pollock fillet. Drizzle each with $1/2$ teaspoon olive oil and sprinkle with salt and pepper. Scatter the mushrooms, lemon zest, basil, and onion on top of each.

Fold the parchment, enclosing the fish, and fold the edges to create an airtight packet. Place the packets on the baking sheets and place the baking sheets in the oven. Bake until the paper puffs up and the fish gives when pressed through the packet, about 10 minutes. Place a packet on each of four plates and serve immediately.

Calories: 157.3 kcal
Fat: 3.6 g
Protein: 23.0 g
Carbohydrates: 8.6 g
Sodium: 340.3 mg

broiled tilapia with fresh herbs, mushrooms, and tomatoes SERVES 4

Olive oil spray, for the baking sheet
3/4 cup fresh basil leaves
3/4 cup fresh parsley leaves
4 garlic cloves
3 tablespoons extra-virgin olive oil
1 tablespoon fresh lime juice
1/8 teaspoon salt
1/4 teaspoon pepper
8 cremini or button mushrooms, each about 2 inches
    across
4 (4-ounce) tilapia fillets, rinsed and patted dry
2 cups grape or cherry tomatoes

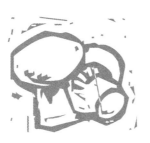

Spray a rimmed baking sheet with olive oil. Arrange a rack 6 inches from the broiler and preheat the broiler to high.

In the work bowl of a food processor, place the basil, parsley, garlic, olive oil, lime juice, and salt and pepper. Process until uniformly chopped and well combined.

Remove the stems from the cremini mushrooms: in one hand, hold a cremini by the cap. With the forefinger and thumb of your other hand, twist the stem off so the hollowed cap is left. Repeat with the remaining mushrooms. Discard the stems (or freeze them for vegetable broth—page 264). Fill each mushroom cap with about $1/4$ teaspoon of the herb mixture. Place them on the prepared baking sheet.

Arrange the tilapia fillets on the baking sheet and spread half of the remaining herb mixture over them. Turn the fillets over and spread the remaining herb mixture over them, making sure that they are completely covered. Scatter the tomatoes on the baking sheet around the fish.

Broil until the fish is firm when pressed and flakes easily, the tomatoes are charred in spots, and the mushrooms are bubbling and soft, about 10 minutes. Place 1 tilapia fillet, 2 mushroom caps, and a few tomatoes on each of four plates and serve.

Calories: 236.7 kcal
Fat: 12.9 g
Protein: 25.3 g
Carbohydrates: 6.6 g
Sodium: 131.8 mg

grilled halibut with fresh berry and ginger salsa

If you have a hard time finding 4-ounce halibut steaks, buy larger steaks and cut them into smaller portions before grilling. SERVES 4

4 cups mixed fresh berries, such as blueberries and
     raspberries
2 tablespoons finely chopped red onion, rinsed and
     drained
1 tablespoon finely chopped crystallized ginger
1 tablespoon apple cider vinegar or fresh lime juice
3/4 teaspoon agave syrup
Salt and ground black pepper
1/8 teaspoon crushed red pepper flakes (optional)
Olive oil spray, for the grill or grill pan
4 (4-ounce) halibut steaks, rinsed and patted dry
1 tablespoon olive oil

In a medium bowl, combine the blueberries, raspberries, onion, ginger, vinegar, agave syrup, $1/8$ teaspoon each salt and pepper, and red pepper flakes, if using. Stir gently to combine and set aside.

If using a gas or charcoal grill, spray the grill grate with olive oil and prepare a medium-hot grill. If using a grill pan, spray it with olive oil and heat over medium-high heat.

Brush both sides of the halibut steaks with the olive oil and season with $1/4$ teaspoon each salt and pepper.

Grill the fish until grill marks are apparent on the underside, 3 to 5 minutes. Turn and grill until the fish is firm when pressed, 3 to 5 minutes.

Divide the berry and candied ginger salsa among four plates. Place a halibut steak on top of or alongside each and serve.

Calories: 263.1 kcal
Fat: 7.3 g
Protein: 31.3 g
Carbohydrates: 21.6 g
Sodium: 259.5 mg

HEALTH BENEFITS:

**Anti-Cancer Heart Healthy Boosts Immunity Boosts Metabolism Improves Digestion
Strong Bones Healthy Skin Miscellaneous**

roasted salmon with pepita and cumin seed crust

Snacking on just one handful of pepitas (pumpkin seeds), about 1 ounce, provides a whopping 9 grams of protein. SERVES 4

1 tablespoon raw pepitas

1 teaspoon cumin seeds

1 teaspoon ground cardamom

1/4 teaspoon salt

4 (4-ounce) wild Alaskan salmon fillets, skin on, rinsed
   and patted dry

2 tablespoons plain nonfat yogurt

2 teaspoons virgin coconut oil

Lemon wedges, for serving

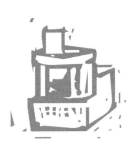

Preheat the oven to 425°F.

Place a small cast-iron or other heavy skillet over medium-high heat. Add the pepitas to the skillet and toast, shaking the pan frequently, until lightly browned, about 4 minutes. Transfer the pepitas to a bowl to cool. Return the skillet to the heat. Place the cumin seeds in the pan and toast shaking the pan frequently, until fragrant, 30 to 45 seconds. Transfer the seeds to a bowl to cool.

In the work bowl of a food processor, place the toasted pepitas and pulse until coarsely chopped. Add the cumin seeds, cardamom, and salt, and pulse two or three times just to combine.

Brush the meaty sides of the salmon fillets with the yogurt. Sprinkle the pepita mixture over the salmon and press to adhere.

Heat a large cast-iron or other ovenproof (not nonstick) skillet over medium-high heat until hot. Add the oil. When the oil is melted, add the salmon, seasoned side down. Cook until the underside is browned, about 3 minutes. Turn the fillets over. Place the skillet in the oven and bake until the salmon is opaque in the center, 3 to 5 minutes, depending on the thickness of the fillets. Serve with lemon wedges.

Calories: 203.0 kcal
Fat: 10.9 g
Protein: 23.6 g
Carbohydrates: 1.5 g
Sodium: 175.5 mg

HEALTH BENEFITS:

**Anti-Cancer Heart Healthy Boosts Immunity Boosts Metabolism Improves Mood
Improves Digestion Strong Bones Healthy Skin**

MASTERING ARTHRITIS

Omega-3s help fight arthritis by easing inflammation. *Eat:* fatty fish such as salmon, sardines, and mackerel; and eat walnuts.

Calcium helps to keep joints limber. *Eat:* low-fat, organic dairy products such as yogurt, kefir, and cottage cheese.

Vitamin C and the antioxidant quercetin work well together to stop pro-inflammatory chemicals from wreaking havoc on your joints. *Eat:* fruits, as well as onions in all shapes and sizes— and don't forget garlic.

Try Poached Salmon with Green Goddess Yogurt (at right).

poached salmon with green goddess yogurt

Try to buy the center cut of the salmon fillet, which will be uniformly thick. Closer to the tail, the fillet gets thinner and narrower and is more likely to cook unevenly. SERVES 8

1 (2-pound) thick wild Alaskan salmon fillet, with skin, rinsed and patted dry
1 1/8 teaspoon salt
3/4 cup nonfat or low-fat plain Greek yogurt
2 anchovies in oil, rinsed, drained, and finely chopped
2 tablespoons chopped scallions (white and green parts) or snipped fresh chives
2 tablespoons chopped parsley
1 tablespoon chopped fresh tarragon
1 garlic clove, minced
1 1/2 teaspoons fresh lemon juice
1 1/2 teaspoons white wine vinegar
1/8 teaspoon ground black pepper
Snipped fresh dill, for garnish
Lemon wedges, for serving

Place the salmon fillet in a pan that is large enough to hold it. Add cold water to cover the fillet by 1 inch and sprinkle 1 teaspoon of the salt over it. Place the pan over high heat and bring to a boil. As soon as the water boils, cover, remove the pan from the heat, and let stand for 10 minutes.

Remove the salmon from the water, drain thoroughly, and place in the refrigerator until chilled, or for up to 8 hours.

Meanwhile, in a small bowl, place the yogurt, anchovies, scallions, parsley, tarragon, garlic, lemon juice, vinegar, remaining 1/8 teaspoon salt, and the pepper. Stir gently until combined. Cover and refrigerate until needed.

Bring the salmon to room temperature before serving. Peel off the skin and place the salmon on a platter. If desired, sprinkle the fresh dill on top and scatter the lemon wedges alongside the fillet. Serve with the green goddess yogurt.

Calories: 168.1 kcal
Fat: 5.3 g
Protein: 27.4 g
Carbohydrates: 1.1 g
Sodium: 505.6 mg

spicy mahi-mahi and mango tacos

SERVES 4

3 tablespoons fresh lime juice

3 tablespoons fresh orange juice

1 garlic clove, chopped

2 teaspoons chili powder

$1/4$ teaspoon salt

$1/4$ teaspoon ground black pepper

$1/8$ teaspoon cayenne pepper

1 pound mahi-mahi, rinsed and patted dry, cut into
bite-size chunks

1 large ripe mango, peeled, pitted, and coarsely
chopped (about 2 cups)

1 tablespoon chopped red onion, rinsed and drained

$1/4$ cup fresh cilantro leaves, chopped

$1/2$ teaspoon seeded, chopped fresh red chile

2 teaspoons virgin coconut oil

4 (8-inch) whole-wheat tortillas

1 ripe avocado, pitted, peeled, and coarsely chopped

Lime wedges, for serving

In a medium bowl, whisk together 2 tablespoons of the lime juice, 2 tablespoons of the orange juice, the garlic, chili powder, salt, black pepper, and cayenne pepper. Add the fish and gently stir to coat. Let stand for at least 10 minutes, or cover and place in the refrigerator for up to 4 hours.

In the meantime, in a medium bowl, combine the mango, onion, cilantro, chile, and remaining 1 tablespoon each lime and orange juice. Stir gently until well combined. Set aside in the refrigerator if you are marinating the fish longer than a few minutes. Let stand at room temperature for at least 20 minutes before serving.

In a large skillet, heat the oil over medium-high heat. Add the fish and its marinade and cook for 3 to 4 minutes, turning frequently, until the fish is opaque.

While the fish cooks, wrap the tortillas in damp paper towels and microwave on high power for 30 seconds.

Gently fold the avocado into the mango mixture.

Divide the fish evenly among the tortillas. Divide the mango mixture among the tacos, spooning it on top of the fish. Serve with lime wedges.

Calories: 405.2 kcal
Fat: 13.9 g
Protein: 26.8 g
Carbohydrates: 43.9 g
Sodium: 409.2 mg

pecan-crusted catfish with cranberry-maple compote

Tangy cranberries and a squeeze of fresh lemon juice are the perfect counterpoints to earthy catfish. Adding half of the maple syrup to the compote after it is cooked allows the syrup's deep flavor to come through. SERVES 4

4 (4-ounce) catfish fillets, rinsed and patted dry
1/2 cup almond milk
6 ounces fresh or frozen cranberries
1/4 cup fresh orange juice
2 tablespoons maple syrup
1 tablespoon olive oil
1 cup (4 ounces) pecans, pulsed in a food processor
    until finely chopped
1/2 teaspoon cayenne pepper
1/4 teaspoon salt
1/4 teaspoon ground black pepper
2 tablespoons nonfat plain yogurt
1 lemon, cut into wedges

In a shallow pan, arrange the catfish fillets in a single layer. Pour the almond milk over the fish. Place in the refrigerator for 30 minutes.

Meanwhile, in a small saucepan, combine the cranberries, orange juice, 1 tablespoon of the maple syrup, and ¼ cup water. Simmer over medium heat until the cranberries have popped and the mixture is saucy, about 15 minutes. Stir in the remaining 1 tablespoon maple syrup and keep warm.

Preheat the oven to 500°F. Brush a baking pan or an ovenproof skillet with the olive oil.

In a medium bowl, combine the pecans, cayenne pepper, salt, and black pepper. Stir well to completely mix. Drain the catfish and pat it dry. Brush the yogurt on both sides of each fillet. One at a time, press both sides of each fish fillet in the nuts, then place in the baking pan or ovenproof skillet.

Bake the fish for 5 minutes. Carefully turn and bake until golden brown on top and cooked through, 6 to 8 minutes. Place a fillet on each of four plates. Spoon the cranberry compote alongside or on top and serve with lemon wedges.

Calories: 462.5 kcal
Fat: 33.4 g
Protein: 24.6 g
Carbohydrates: 19.4 g
Sodium: 226.7 mg

**Anti-Cancer Heart Healthy Boosts Immunity Boosts Metabolism Improves Digestion
Strong Bones Healthy Skin**

almond-orange rainbow trout
with chipotle yogurt sauce SERVES 4

FOR THE RAINBOW TROUT
Olive oil spray, for the baking sheet
$1/3$ cup (1 ounce) sliced almonds
1 slice whole-wheat bread, torn into pieces
1 garlic clove, finely chopped
Grated zest of 1 orange
$1/8$ teaspoon cayenne pepper
4 (4-ounce) rainbow trout fillets, rinsed and patted dry
$1/8$ teaspoon salt
$1/4$ teaspoon ground black pepper
1 tablespoon nonfat plain yogurt

FOR THE CHIPOTLE YOGURT SAUCE
1 chipotle chile in adobo sauce, seeded and chopped,
      plus $1/2$ teaspoon adobo sauce
3 garlic cloves, finely chopped
Juice of 1 lemon, plus more to taste
2 tablespoons fresh orange juice
$1/2$ cup low-fat plain Greek yogurt

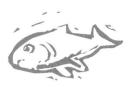

Preheat the oven to 400°F. Spray a baking sheet with olive oil.

Begin the fish. In the work bowl of a food processor, place the almonds, bread, garlic, orange zest, and cayenne pepper. Pulse several times until roughly chopped. Pour the mixture onto a shallow plate.

Prepare the Chipotle Yogurt Sauce. In the work bowl of a food processor, combine the chile and adobo sauce, garlic, lemon juice, and orange juice. Blend to a smooth paste. Transfer to a small bowl. Add the low-fat yogurt and stir until combined. Taste and add more lemon juice, if desired. Set aside.

Season the trout with the salt and pepper. Brush the top of each fillet with the nonfat yogurt. Press the yogurt-coated side of each fillet into the almond mixture. Place the fillets nut side up on the prepared baking sheet.

Bake until the fish is firm and not translucent when you slide a thin-bladed knife in to peek at the center, about 10 minutes.

Spoon the sauce onto four plates. Place a piece of trout on top of each and serve.

Calories: 232.1 kcal
Fat: 9.8 g
Protein: 25.3 g
Carbohydrates: 10.9 g
Sodium: 500.9 mg

broiled mackerel with lemon-caper vinaigrette SERVES 4

SAFELY COOKING MEAT, POULTRY, AND FISH

The recipes in this book give you good signs to look for to determine whether the meat, poultry, or fish is cooked. Where necessary, the recipes make allowances for the fact that the internal temperature of cooked food continues to rise 5° to 10°F off the heat. But when you're cooking without a good recipe, the best way to know if meat, poultry, and fish are cooked properly is to use a thermometer. The USDA recommends cooking meat and poultry to the following internal temperatures:

Steaks and roasts—145°F

Fish—145°F

Pork—160°F

Ground beef—160°F

Egg dishes—160°F

Chicken breasts—165°F

Whole poultry—165°F

Olive oil spray, for the baking sheet
Pinch of grated lemon zest
2 teaspoons fresh lemon juice
1 teaspoon champagne vinegar
$1/4$ teaspoon honey
$1/4$ teaspoon Dijon mustard
1 tablespoon drained nonpareil capers
1 tablespoon minced parsley
1 small garlic clove, finely chopped
$1/4$ teaspoon salt
$1/4$ teaspoon ground black pepper
2 tablespoons plus 2 teaspoons extra-virgin olive oil
4 (4-ounce) mackerel fillets, skin on, rinsed and patted dry
1 bunch watercress, rinsed

Place a rack 6 inches from the broiler and preheat the broiler to high. Spray a rimmed baking sheet with olive oil.

In a small bowl, combine the lemon zest and juice, vinegar, honey, mustard, capers, parsley, garlic, and salt and pepper. Whisk together thoroughly. Whisking constantly, slowly drizzle in 2 tablespoons of the olive oil. Set aside.

Using a sharp knife, make three slashes in the skin of each mackerel fillet. Lightly brush the fillets with the remaining 2 teaspoons olive oil and arrange them skin side up on the prepared baking sheet. Broil until the fish is cooked through, about 5 minutes.

Divide the watercress among four serving plates. Place one fillet on top of each serving of watercress, and divide the sauce among the plates, drizzling it over the mackerel. Serve.

Calories: 349.9 kcal
Fat: 26.8 g
Protein: 24.6 g
Carbohydrates: 1.8 g
Sodium: 294.7 mg

grilled sardines with lemon and basil SERVES 4

Olive oil spray, for the grill or grill pan
12 (2 to 3 ounces each) fresh sardines, cleaned, heads
    and tails intact
1/2 teaspoon salt
12 fresh basil leaves
12 strips lemon zest removed with a vegetable peeler,
    plus 1 lemon, sliced in wedges, for serving
1 tablespoon extra-virgin olive oil

If grilling on a gas or charcoal grill, spray the grill grate with the olive oil and prepare a medium-hot grill. If using a grill pan, spray it with olive oil and heat over medium-high heat.

Rinse the sardines inside and out and pat them dry. In the body cavity of each sardine sprinkle a little salt and place 1 basil leaf and 1 strip of lemon zest. Fold the sardines closed and brush them on both sides with the olive oil.

Grill the sardines until just cooked through, turning once, 4 to 5 minutes. Serve with lemon wedges.

Calories: 124.3 kcal
Fat: 7.1 g
Protein: 10.9 g
Carbohydrates: 0.8 g
Sodium: 459.9 mg

linguine with anchovies, garlic, and parsley SERVES 4

8 ounces whole-wheat linguine
2 tablespoons extra-virgin olive oil
8 anchovy fillets, rinsed and drained
4 garlic cloves, coarsely chopped
$1/4$ teaspoon crushed red pepper flakes
1 cup parsley leaves, coarsely chopped
$1/4$ teaspoon salt
$1/4$ teaspoon ground black pepper

Bring a large pot of water to a boil. Cook the linguine according to package directions.

About 2 minutes before the pasta is cooked, heat the olive oil over medium heat in a large skillet. Add the anchovies and cook, crushing and stirring them with a wooden spoon, until the anchovies are falling apart, about 1 minute. Stir in the garlic and red pepper flakes and cook until fragrant, another 30 seconds.

When the linguine is ready, drain it and add it to the skillet along with the parsley, salt, and black pepper. Use two wooden spoons to toss the linguine and thoroughly coat it with the sauce. Serve.

Calories: 290.4 kcal
Fat: 9.4 g
Protein: 12.0 g
Carbohydrates: 41.1 g
Sodium: 432.4 mg

coconut-curry steamed mussels

Serve with steamed brown rice (page 261) or quinoa (page 262) for a filling dinner and a great way of soaking up all the coconut-curry sauce! SERVES 4

2 pounds mussels
2 teaspoons virgin coconut oil
$^1/_2$ cup finely chopped red onion
2 garlic cloves, minced
2 teaspoons finely chopped fresh ginger
1 tablespoon curry powder
$^1/_2$ cup coconut milk
2 tablespoons chopped fresh cilantro

MASTERING FISH AND SHELLFISH: SMART STORAGE

- Fish and shellfish should be refrigerated only for a few hours. Wrap tightly in plastic and place in the refrigerator in a shallow pan filled with ice. Simply refrigerating raw seafood will not keep it from spoiling. It must be frozen or eaten fresh.
- Do not put unwrapped fish directly on ice, as the water may flush out some of its flavor.
- Defrost frozen seafood in the refrigerator just before eating. Do not thaw in the microwave; this will ruin its texture.
- Store live mollusks in your refrigerator in a container that is covered loosely with a clean, damp cloth.

Rinse the mussels under cold running water. Pull out any "beards" by wiggling them gently and then pulling down toward the pointed end of the mussel. Discard any mussels with cracked shells or that do not close when gently tapped on the counter.

In a Dutch oven or other large, deep pot, heat the oil over medium heat. Add the onion, garlic, and ginger and cook, stirring occasionally, for 3 minutes. Add the curry powder and cook, stirring, for 30 seconds. Reduce the heat to low. Add $^1/_2$ cup water and simmer for 1 minute.

Add the cleaned mussels and increase the heat to medium. Cover the pan and simmer, gently shaking the pan from time to time, until the mussels open, 4 to 5 minutes. Use a slotted spoon to transfer the mussels to a large serving bowl (discard any that did not open) and cover to keep warm.

Bring the cooking liquid to a boil and simmer 3 to 4 minutes, until slightly reduced and thickened. Stir in the coconut milk and cook for 2 minutes more. Stir in the cilantro and pour the sauce around and over the mussels. Serve.

Calories: 232.1 kcal
Fat: 12.2 g
Protein: 20.1 g
Carbohydrates: 10.3 g
Sodium: 466.0 mg

mussels with linguine SERVES 6

12 ounces whole-wheat linguine

2 pounds mussels

1 tablespoon olive oil

^{1}/$_4$ cup finely chopped shallots

1 garlic clove, finely chopped

1 tablespoon tomato paste

1 pound plum tomatoes, cored and cut into
 ^{1}/$_4$-inch cubes

^{1}/$_2$ cup chopped mixed fresh herbs, such as basil,
 parsley, marjoram, and /or thyme

^{1}/$_4$ cup pitted oil-cured black olives, coarsely chopped

1 fresh or dried bay leaf (optional)

^{1}/$_4$ teaspoon ground black pepper

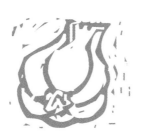

Bring a large pot of water to a boil. Stir in the linguine and cook according to package directions. Drain.

Meanwhile, rinse the mussels under cold running water. Pull out any "beards" by wiggling them gently and then pulling down toward the pointed end of the mussel. Discard any mussels with cracked shells or that do not close when gently tapped on the counter.

In a Dutch oven or other large, deep pot, heat the olive oil over medium heat. Add the shallots and garlic and cook, stirring occasionally, until softened, about 3 minutes. Stir in the tomato paste and cook for 1 minute. Stir in the tomatoes, herbs, olives, and bay leaf, if using, and bring to a simmer. Cover and simmer gently for 5 minutes.

Remove the lid and stir the tomato mixture. Add the mussels, cover, and simmer, gently shaking the pan from time to time, until the mussels open, 4 to 5 minutes. Use a slotted spoon to transfer the mussels to a serving bowl (discard any that did not open) and keep warm. Stir the pepper into the broth and taste. If the broth is a little thin, turn up the heat and simmer until the sauce is reduced and flavorful, 3 to 5 minutes. Discard the bay leaf.

Divide the linguine among six serving plates or bowls. Top with the mussels and tomato-herb broth. Serve immediately.

Calories: 343.3 kcal
Fat: 7.0 g
Protein: 22.8 g
Carbohydrates: 48.3 g
Sodium: 391.9 mg

bay scallops with toasted sesame seeds SERVES 4

2 tablespoons olive oil
1 pound farmed bay scallops
$1/4$ teaspoon salt
$1/4$ teaspoon ground pepper
1 teaspoon fresh lemon juice
$1/4$ teaspoon toasted sesame oil
2 tablespoons white or black sesame seeds, or a
    combination, toasted (page 96)
Lemon wedges, for serving

In a well-seasoned cast-iron skillet big enough to hold the scallops in a single layer, heat the olive oil over medium-high heat until hot but not smoking. Add the scallops and cook, shaking the pan occasionally, until lightly browned, 2 to 3 minutes.

Sprinkle the scallops with the salt and pepper, and add $1/4$ cup water to the pan. Cook, scraping up any browned bits, until saucy. Stir in the lemon juice and sesame oil. Transfer to a serving platter and sprinkle with the sesame seeds. Serve with lemon wedges.

Calories: 198.0 kcal
Fat: 10.3 g
Protein: 19.8 g
Carbohydrates: 4.5 g
Sodium: 302.8 mg

MASTERING FISH AND SHELLFISH: SMART PREPARATION

Fish

- Fish can be very simple to prepare if you buy it already filleted or cut into steaks.
- Before cooking, be sure to rinse in cold water and pat dry.
- Broiling, poaching, and searing are the healthiest ways to prepare fish, followed by grilling and steaming. Try to avoid sautéing and frying whenever possible.

Shellfish

- Rinse under cold water, scrub lightly, and pat dry.
- I am a big believer in shelling and deveining your shrimp. The shrimp's intestine runs the length of the shrimp along the back of its shell. Take a small knife and make a slit about $1/8$ inch deep along the back of the shrimp, and scrape out the gunk. This will help you to avoid potential food poisoning.
- Cook gently, as they are quick to burn and easily overcooked, which damages their nutrients.

Mollusks

- At home, give whole oysters a quick scrub under running water. Discard any with cracked shells.
- Mollusks are extremely prone to contamination, so it's always best to eat them fully cooked.
- If you choose to boil them, shells will open during boiling. After the shells open, continue to boil for 3 to 5 more minutes. If steaming, cook for 4 to 9 minutes in total.
- Use small pots to boil or steam shellfish. If too many shells are cooking in the same pot, it's possible that those in the middle won't get thoroughly cooked. *Discard any clams, mussels, or oysters that do not open during cooking.* Closed shells may mean they have not received adequate heat.
- If cooking shucked oysters, boil or simmer for at least 3 minutes, or bake for at least 10 minutes at 450°F.

chili-lime shrimp skewers with pineapple-mint salsa SERVES 4

Olive oil spray, for the grill or grill pan

3 tablespoons fresh lime juice

2 tablespoons olive oil

1 1/4 pounds large shrimp, peeled and deveined

1 pineapple

2 tablespoons finely chopped red onion, rinsed and
    drained

1/4 cup packed fresh mint, chopped

1/4 to 1/2 teaspoon seeded and minced fresh red chile

1 teaspoon chili powder

1/2 teaspoon salt

1/4 teaspoon ground black pepper

If using a gas or charcoal grill, spray the grill with olive oil and prepare a medium-hot grill. If using a grill pan, spray it with olive oil and heat over medium-high heat.

Place 8 skewers in a pan of water; let stand for at least 20 minutes.

In a medium bowl, whisk together 2 tablespoons of the lime juice and the olive oil. Add the shrimp and stir to coat. Let stand for 15 minutes.

Use a serrated knife to cut the top off the pineapple. Cut a thin slice from the bottom and stand the pineapple upright on a cutting board. Beginning at the top, use a gentle sawing motion to cut down the length of the pineapple and remove a strip of the rough skin; try to cut deep enough that you remove most of the "eyes." Repeat all the way around the pineapple until the skin is removed. Use a paring knife to remove any remaining "eyes." Lay the pineapple on its side and carefully cut it crosswise into 1/2-inch slices.

Grill the pineapple slices just until tender, about 4 minutes per side. Transfer to a work surface. Cut the pineapple into 1/2-inch pieces, discarding the tough center of each slice; you should have about 4 cups. Place the pineapple in a medium bowl and add the onion, mint, chile, and remaining 1 tablespoon lime juice. Stir gently and set aside.

Pat the shrimp dry and thread them on the skewers. Sprinkle with the chili powder, salt, and pepper. Grill until just opaque in the center, 4 to 5 minutes, turning once. Serve with the pineapple-mint salsa.

Calories: 234.9 kcal
Fat: 8.5 g
Protein: 23.4 g
Carbohydrates: 17.1 g
Sodium: 490.0 mg

ginger shrimp rolls with green papaya slaw SERVES 6

FOR THE SHRIMP

$1/4$ cup rice wine or dry sherry

2 tablespoons low-sodium tamari

1 teaspoon toasted sesame oil

1 teaspoon honey

1 tablespoon minced fresh ginger

Grated zest of 1 lime

$1^1/4$ pounds medium shrimp, peeled and deveined

FOR THE GREEN PAPAYA SLAW

1 pound green papaya (about half of a medium-large
    papaya), peeled and seeded

3 tablespoons rice vinegar

1 tablespoon honey

Pinch of crushed red pepper flakes

FOR THE LIME SAUCE

Juice of 2 limes (about $1/4$ cup)

1 tablespoon honey

1 tablespoon Asian fish sauce (nam pla or nuac mam)

1 teaspoon grated fresh ginger

1 garlic clove, minced

$1/4$ teaspoon crushed red pepper flakes

1 tablespoon sesame seeds

2 heads butterhead lettuce, leaves separated

Prepare the shrimp. In a large bowl, mix the rice wine, tamari, oil, honey, ginger, and lime zest. Add the shrimp, toss to coat well, and place in the refrigerator for at least 15 minutes and up to 1 hour.

Meanwhile, prepare the slaw. Using a food processor fitted with the grating attachment or using the large holes on a box grater, grate the green papaya; you should have about 4 cups. Transfer to a medium bowl. In a small bowl, whisk together the vinegar, honey, and red pepper flakes. Pour over the grated papaya and toss well to combine. Set aside.

Prepare the sauce. In a small bowl, place the lime juice, honey, fish sauce, ginger, garlic, and red pepper flakes. Whisk to combine and set aside.

Place a large skillet over medium heat. Add the sesame seeds and toast until fragrant and lightly browned, 2 to 3 minutes. Immediately transfer the seeds to a plate. Place the skillet over medium-high heat. Add the shrimp to the skillet with $1/4$ cup of the marinade and bring to a simmer. Cook until the shrimp are slightly firm, 4 to 5 minutes, turning once.

To form a roll, place a lettuce leaf on the work surface. Place 2 shrimp in the leaf and top with about 3 tablespoons of the slaw. Drizzle with about $1/2$ teaspoon sauce and sprinkle with a few sesame seeds. Repeat until all the shrimp are used. Divide the rolls evenly among six plates and serve.

Calories: 160.0 kcal
Fat: 2.5 g
Protein: 17.1 g
Carbohydrates: 15.5 g
Sodium: 600.8 mg

calamari with salsa verde and arugula SERVES 4

$2/3$ cup parsley leaves

2 tablespoons sliced scallions (white and green parts)

2 tablespoons drained capers

2 anchovy fillets, rinsed and drained

1 garlic clove, coarsely chopped, plus 3 garlic cloves, chopped

$1/4$ teaspoon ground black pepper

2 tablespoons extra-virgin olive oil

6 cups arugula, shredded if the leaves are large

1 pound cleaned squid tubes, cut crosswise into $1/4$-inch-wide rings, rinsed and patted dry

In the work bowl of a food processor, place the parsley, scallions, capers, anchovies, 1 garlic clove, the pepper, and 1 tablespoon of the olive oil. Process until uniformly chopped and well combined, scraping down the sides of the work bowl once or twice. Set the salsa aside.

Divide the arugula among four plates.

In a large skillet, heat the remaining 1 tablespoon olive oil over medium heat. Add the 3 remaining garlic cloves and cook for 30 seconds. Add the calamari and spread in a single layer. Turn the heat to medium-high and cook without stirring until the calamari are golden on the bottom, about 4 minutes.

Stir in the salsa and cook for 1 minute. Pour the warm calamari and salsa mixture on top of the arugula. Let stand for 4 to 5 minutes to slightly wilt the arugula before serving.

Calories: 189.4 kcal

Fat: 9.1 g

Protein: 19.7 g

Carbohydrates: 6.7 g

Sodium: 265.5 mg

vegetarian main dishes

MEDITERRANEAN PIZZA

ROASTED OR GRILLED VEGETABLES WITH ROMESCO SAUCE

FRITTATA WITH SPINACH, POTATOES, PEPPERS, AND FETA

SPINACH AND RED ONION QUICHE

CHARD POTSTICKERS WITH TAMARI DIPPING SAUCE

VEGETABLE STIR-FRY WITH LEMONGRASS

ALMOND AND VEGETABLE PAD THAI

LINGUINE WITH ZUCCHINI, GRAPE TOMATOES, AND CREAMY LEMON-YOGURT SAUCE

BARLEY RISOTTO WITH ASPARAGUS AND LEMON

WINTER VEGETABLE COUSCOUS

QUINOA-STUFFED PEPPERS

BLACK BEAN CHILI

BAKED RATATOUILLE WITH PARMESAN

mediterranean pizza SERVES 4

1 to 2 tablespoons organic cornmeal, for the baking
    sheet
4 cups (packed) shredded spinach (about 5 ounces)
Whole-wheat flour, for work surface
1 pound whole-wheat pizza dough, thawed if frozen
2 teaspoons extra-virgin olive oil
4 plum tomatoes, thinly sliced
1 tablespoon coarsely chopped fresh marjoram,
    oregano, or basil leaves
$1/2$ small red onion, thinly sliced
$1/3$ cup crumbled low-fat feta cheese
$1/4$ cup pitted kalamata olives, coarsely chopped
$1/2$ teaspoon ground black pepper

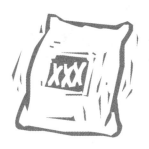

Preheat the oven to 450°F. Spread the cornmeal on a large baking sheet; alternatively, rub the baking sheet with olive oil.

Place the spinach in a microwave-safe bowl with a lid. Cover and microwave on high power until the spinach is bright green and wilted, about 1 minute. Transfer to a strainer and rinse with cold water. When cool enough to handle, wrap the leaves in a clean kitchen towel and squeeze out all of the excess liquid. Remove the spinach from the towel, using your fingers to loosen and separate the leaves. Set aside.

On a lightly floured work surface, use a rolling pin and your hands to roll and stretch the dough to a roughly 10 by 14-inch rectangle; if the dough becomes so elastic that after it is rolled it just snaps back, contracting to its original size, let it rest for a few minutes before continuing to roll. Transfer the dough to the prepared baking sheet.

Brush the dough with 1 teaspoon of the olive oil. Arrange the tomatoes on the dough. Sprinkle the marjoram over the tomatoes. Spread the spinach on top, followed by the onion, feta, olives, and pepper. Drizzle the remaining 1 teaspoon olive oil over the pie.

Bake until the crust is golden, 15 to 20 minutes.

Calories: 388.5 kcal
Fat: 10.3 g
Protein: 13.8 g
Carbohydrates: 59.9 g
Sodium: 814.1 mg

MASTERING VEGETABLES
Smart Selection
- A darker color is always better. The darker the color, the more nutrients. Choose red onions over white, black olives over green. Also, pick the tomato with the redder hue, the eggplant that is a darker shade of purple, the greener type of lettuce—you get the idea.
- Try to get fresh vegetables that have ripened on the vine, not in transit. This allows the food to fully develop its flavor and nutrient content.
- When vegetables are picked they have a reserve of protective nutrients. The longer the time between a vegetable's having been picked and its landing on your table, the lesser its nutritional value. The reserved nutrients are utilized to protect the fruit or vegetable from oxidizing or spoiling; this is why proper storage is one of the keys to maximizing the nutrients in your produce.

Smart Storage
- Most vegetables should be refrigerated in a storage bin or storage bags for optimal retention of nutrients and eaten within 2 to 4 days.
- The following vegetables must be stored at room temperature in a dry, dark place: eggplant, tomato, garlic, squash, any kind of potato, onions, and avocado. Refrigeration destroys the nutrients in these foods. Only refrigerate them if they have been cut, and then be sure to eat them within 24 hours.

Smart Preparation

- Cut veggies into small pieces so as to not overcook them; overcooking kills their nutritional value. On the other hand, raw food isn't the way to go either, as the nutrients in most vegetables are more available to your body when the vegetables are cooked properly. Many of us don't have the digestive enzymes for raw vegetables, so they can upset our stomachs. By cooking them we soften their fiber, making them easier to digest and allowing their healthful nutrients to become more readily absorbed. For example, spinach has more available vitamin K when cooked, corn has more vitamin C, carrots more beta-carotene, tomatoes more available lycopene, and so on.

- Grilling, baking, roasting, sautéing, and microwaving are all great ways to prepare your veggies. Boiling and stovetop steaming are less than ideal because some of the nutrients can be lost into the water.

- Timing when cooking vegetables is essential for maximizing nutritional benefits. Most vegetables should cook for 3 to 7 minutes. When sautéing vegetables on their own, follow these simple guidelines (see page 216 for more ways to prepare vegetables):

Sauté for 3 minutes	Peas, summer squash, tomatoes
Sauté for 5 minutes	Cauliflower, broccoli, kale, brussels sprouts, carrots, asparagus, cabbage
Sauté for 7 minutes	Bell peppers, onions, leeks, mushrooms

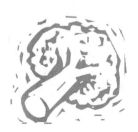

roasted or grilled vegetables with romesco sauce SERVES 6

Olive oil spray, if grilling

6 plum tomatoes (about 1 pound), cored and halved

3 medium zucchini, sliced in half lengthwise

4 bell peppers, 1 red and the rest red, yellow, or orange, cored, seeded, and each cut into 6 wedges

2 small eggplants (about 6 ounces each), each cut lengthwise into 3 slices

1 pound asparagus, ends trimmed

1 pound large cremini or button mushrooms, stemmed

1 large red onion, cut crosswise into $1/4$-inch slices

5 tablespoons extra-virgin olive oil

$3/4$ teaspoon salt

$1^1/4$ teaspoons ground black pepper

$1/2$ cup slivered almonds, toasted (page 96)

6 garlic cloves, peeled

2 tablespoons sherry vinegar

If roasting the vegetables, preheat the oven to 450°F and have ready three or four large, rimmed baking sheets or shallow roasting pans and one pan or small cast-iron skillet for the mushrooms. If grilling, spray a grill grate with olive oil and prepare a medium-hot grill.

Place half of the vegetables in a large bowl and add $1^1/2$ tablespoons of the olive oil, $1/4$ teaspoon of the salt, and $1/2$ teaspoon of the pepper. Use your hands to gently toss the vegetables so that they are evenly coated with oil. Repeat with the remaining vegetables and another $1^1/2$ tablespoons olive oil, $1/4$ teaspoon salt, and $1/2$ teaspoon pepper.

If roasting, arrange the vegetables on the baking sheets, placing the mushrooms in their own small pan. Do not overcrowd the vegetables, or they will steam instead of roasting. Roast until lightly browned and tender when pierced with the tip of a sharp knife, 20 to 40 minutes. Some vegetables may be done before others, so start checking after 20 minutes of roasting, and remove any vegetables that are ready. Return the remaining vegetables to the oven until they are fully roasted.

Or grill the vegetables 5 to 6 minutes per side.

When the vegetables are cooked, set aside 4 tomato halves and 6 red bell pepper wedges. Arrange the remaining vegetables on a large platter; set aside while you prepare the sauce.

In the work bowl of a food processor, place the almonds and garlic. Process until the nuts are ground. Add the reserved tomatoes and bell peppers along with the remaining 2 tablespoons olive oil, the remaining 1/4 teaspoon each salt and pepper, and the vinegar. Process until the mixture is well combined; it will not be completely smooth. Transfer to a small bowl and serve with the vegetables.

.Calories: 283.4 kcal
Fat: 18.3 g
Protein: 9.5 g
Carbohydrates: 26.0 g
Sodium: 264.7 mg

frittata with spinach, potatoes, peppers, and feta

A well-seasoned cast-iron skillet is the best choice for cooking frittatas. Not only does it increase the iron content in the dish, but it also makes getting the slices out of the pan very easy.

SERVES 4

2 cups baby spinach leaves or coarsely chopped flat-leaf spinach, rinsed
1 tablespoon olive oil
1 cup diced red onion
Pinch of salt
3 ounces cremini or button mushrooms, trimmed and sliced (about 1 cup)
1 small (about 3 ounces) russet potato, cut into 1/4-inch cubes (about 1/2 cup)
1/2 red bell pepper, cut into 1/4-inch cubes (about 3/4 cup)
4 large eggs
1/2 cup crumbled low-fat feta cheese
1 teaspoon chopped fresh oregano leaves
1/4 teaspoon ground black pepper

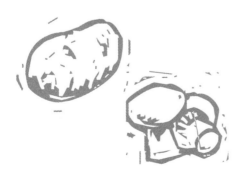

Set a rack about 4 inches from the broiler and preheat the broiler to low.

Heat an 8- to 10-inch cast-iron or other ovenproof (not nonstick) skillet over low heat. Add the spinach with the rinse water still clinging to the leaves (if the spinach is completely dry, add a tablespoon of water to the pan with the spinach). Cover and cook until the leaves have barely wilted, about 1 minute. Transfer to a colander and use tongs to squeeze out as much liquid as possible. Wipe the skillet clean.

Add the olive oil to the cleaned skillet and heat over medium heat. Add the onion and salt and cook, stirring occasionally, until the onion is beginning to soften, about 2 minutes. Add the mushrooms and cook, stirring occasionally, until lightly browned, about 2 minutes. Stir in the potato and pepper, cover, and cook, stirring once or twice, until the potato is tender but still firm, another 5 to 7 minutes.

Meanwhile, in a medium bowl, whisk the eggs until lightly beaten. Stir in the reserved spinach, the feta, oregano, and black pepper. When the potato mixture is cooked, evenly pour the egg mixture over it. Cook until the eggs are set around the edges, about 10 minutes.

Place the skillet under the broiler for 1 to 2 minutes, until the top of the frittata is puffed and lightly browned. Serve hot.

Calories: 197.8 kcal
Fat: 11.2 g
Protein: 14.0 g
Carbohydrates: 12.3 g
Sodium: 510.8 mg

spinach and red onion quiche

SERVES 6

1 frozen whole-wheat piecrust, set at room
   temperature for 20 minutes
1 tablespoon olive oil
1/2 medium red onion, thinly sliced
1/4 teaspoon salt
1/4 teaspoon ground black pepper
1 garlic clove, finely chopped
4 ounces shiitake mushrooms, stems trimmed and
   discarded, caps thinly sliced
1 pound fresh spinach, trimmed and coarsely chopped
3 large eggs
3/4 cup almond milk
1/2 cup grated Parmesan cheese
Pinch of freshly grated nutmeg

Preheat the oven to 350°F.

Use a fork to prick the piecrust in several places to prevent bubbles. Bake until lightly browned, about 20 minutes. Remove from the oven and set aside.

Meanwhile, in a large skillet, heat the olive oil over medium-low heat. Add the onion and $1/8$ teaspoon each salt and pepper, and cook, stirring occasionally, until softened, about 4 minutes. Add the garlic and cook until fragrant and lightly browned, about 30 seconds. Add the mushrooms and cook until softened, about 4 minutes. Add the spinach to the skillet and cook until wilted, 1 to 2 minutes.

Transfer the spinach mixture to a colander. Press firmly with the back of a spoon to squeeze out as much liquid as possible. Transfer the spinach mixture to the crust and spread to cover. Place the crust pan on a rimmed baking sheet, if desired, to make it easier to transfer the quiche to the oven.

In a medium bowl, whisk together the eggs, almond milk, Parmesan, nutmeg, and remaining $1/8$ teaspoon each salt and pepper. Pour the egg mixture over the spinach. Bake until the quiche is just set when the pan is gently nudged, 40 to 45 minutes. Let stand for 15 minutes before serving.

Calories: 290.2 kcal
Fat: 19.3 g
Protein: 11.1 g
Carbohydrates: 20.2 g
Sodium: 465.9 mg

GOING ORGANIC DOESN'T HAVE TO BE EXPENSIVE—REALLY!

Here are some cost-saving tips that anyone can use.

- **Buy fruits and veggies in season.** They are cheaper and better for the environment.
- **Grow your own vegetables.** This is an obvious one. You can produce up to 100 pounds of food a year in a 6 by 6-foot raised bed in your backyard. It's all natural and nearly free.
- **Frequent local farmers' markets.** Because there are minimal costs for transport, packaging, and advertising, you pay less.
- **Clip coupons.** In the past, coupons for organics have been hard to come by, but that is changing. Now that many big-box stores such as Safeway and Walmart are starting their own organic lines, coupons are more readily available. Here is a great Web site dedicated to saving you money when shopping organic: www.organicgrocerydeals.com.
- **Buy frozen.** Organic produce retains the majority of its flavor and nutrients whether it is fresh or frozen, so don't be afraid to save a few bucks by shopping in the freezer section.
- **Buy in bulk.** Buying in bulk is significantly cheaper. Use the bins at health food stores and farmers' markets for grains, nuts, legumes, and cereals.
- **Eat less meat.** We don't need to eat the amount of meat we do. Instead of eating crappy meat all week long, replace it with bean-, grain-, and plant-based meals—save your dough for the good stuff. A grass-fed steak once a week is plenty.
- **Shop online.** Often, organics are cheaper online because you are not paying for an expensive storefront. The GreenPeople directory from the Organic Consumers Association (www.organicconsumers.org/purelink.html) is a good place to begin your online search for affordable foods. For a list of cyber-markets offering organic products in your area, go to www.organickitchen.com.
- **Prioritize your grocery budget.** Free up more dollars for organic food by trimming the fat from your conventional food budget. Examine and reassign the dollars you spend every month at drive-thrus, on coffee drinks, bagels, and even trips to vending machines. A small change in your eating habits could free up the money you need to buy the organic foods you really want. Do your homework ahead of time and shop smart.
- **Comparison shop.** There are many resources and locales for buying organics. Do your homework on who offers the best deals. For example, in some areas currently, organic milk at Trader Joe's is nearly $2 cheaper than that offered at Whole Foods.
- **Buy a share in a community-supported agriculture program (CSA).** When you buy a share in a CSA, you pay a portion of a local farm's operating expenses. In return, you receive weekly boxes of fresh fruits and vegetables at a cost of $300 to $500 for a 24- to 26-week growing season. Many CSAs accept monthly payments, and you may be able to

buy a half-share or save even more money by actually helping out on the farm every now and then! Check the Web sites of government and nonprofit organizations such as the Alternative Farming Systems Information Center (afsic.nal.usda.gov); FoodRoutes (www .foodroutes.org); and LocalHarvest (www.localharvest.org) to find a CSA near you.

- **Join a co-op.** A food cooperative is a member-owned business that provides groceries and other products to its members at a discount. Most of the products are organic and come from local family farms. All you do is sign up and pay some dues. Co-op members who volunteer to work may get additional discounts on any products they buy. To find a co-op near you, check out the food co-op directory on the Web site of the online magazine the Cooperative Grocer (www.cooperativegrocer.coop/coops). If there's no co-op in your area, and you've got the time and desire to do so, you can start your own. The Cooperative Grocers' Information Network (www.cgin.coop) has a brochure to show you how.

- **Join a buying club.** Buying-club members purchase organic food and products in bulk and then split the stash—saving as much as 30 to 40 percent off retail price. Ask a co-op near you about starting a buying club with your friends and neighbors. Or, ask a local natural food store where they get their goods and then contact the distributor directly.

- **Not everything has to be organic.** You don't have to buy organic versions of every single food item to make a difference in your health or the planet's. Absolutely buy organic beef and dairy. Replace dairy items you can't afford with almond-, rice-, or coconut-milk alternatives. Buy organic poultry and eggs whenever possible.

As for produce, it is not all created equal when it comes to pesticides. The nonprofit Environmental Working Group (www.ewg.org) has compiled a list of the produce that carries the most and the least pesticide residue. These "clean 15" have the least pesticide residue (listed starting with least pesticides): onions, avocados, frozen sweet corn, pineapples, mangos, asparagus, frozen sweet peas, kiwi fruit, cabbages, eggplants, papayas, watermelons, broccoli, tomatoes, and sweet potatoes. The following "dirty dozen" have the most pesticide residue and you should buy only the organics (listed starting with the most pesticides): peaches, apples, sweet bell peppers, celery, nectarines, strawberries, cherries, kale, lettuce, imported grapes (domestic grapes are better, but not great), carrots, and pears.

If you don't have this list handy when you're shopping, use this as a general guideline: thick-skinned fruits and veggies don't need to be organic. Eat citrus fruits, melons, bananas, and kiwi instead of berries, peaches, and apples if you can't afford organic versions. You can peel the skin off thin-skinned nonorganic fruits and veggies, but you will lose a lot of good fiber and nutrients the skin holds. Always rinse your produce before eating or cooking it.

chard potstickers with tamari dipping sauce MAKES ABOUT 3 DOZEN; SERVES 6

FOR THE DIPPING SAUCE
$1/3$ cup low-sodium tamari
$1/3$ cup rice wine vinegar
1 teaspoon toasted sesame oil
$1/2$ teaspoon grated fresh ginger
Pinch of crushed red pepper flakes

FOR THE POTSTICKERS
2 tablespoons plus 1 teaspoon virgin coconut oil
8 ounces Swiss chard, leaves chopped, stems minced
3 ounces shiitake mushrooms, trimmed, caps finely
    chopped
2 scallions (white and green parts), thinly sliced
2 garlic cloves, minced
2 teaspoons minced fresh ginger
$1/4$ teaspoon crushed red pepper flakes
2 tablespoons chopped fresh cilantro
2 teaspoons rice wine vinegar
1 teaspoon toasted sesame oil
1 teaspoon low-sodium tamari
$1/4$ teaspoon salt
$1/4$ teaspoon ground black pepper
About 3 dozen round dumpling wrappers

Prepare the dipping sauce. In a small bowl, combine the tamari, vinegar, sesame oil, ginger, and red pepper flakes. Stir and set aside.

Prepare the filling. In a large skillet, heat 1 teaspoon of the coconut oil over medium heat. Add the chard, mushrooms, scallions, garlic, ginger, and red pepper flakes, and cook, stirring constantly, until the chard stems are tender but still crisp and any liquid has evaporated, 3 to 4 minutes. Use tongs to squeeze any excess liquid from the chard and transfer it to a medium bowl. Stir in the cilantro, vinegar, sesame oil, tamari, salt, and pepper.

Shape the potstickers. Have a ramekin of water ready and a baking sheet lined with parchment or wax paper. Work with 1 wrapper at a time and keep the rest covered with a damp kitchen towel to prevent them from drying out.

If using a potsticker press, place a wrapper in the press. Spoon 1 teaspoon of filling into the center of the wrapper. Use your finger or a small brush to moisten half of the edge with water. Fold the press over, and press to crimp and seal. Set aside on the prepared baking sheet and cover with a damp towel.

If not using a press, lay 1 wrapper on a work surface and spoon 1 teaspoon of filling in the center of the wrapper. Use your finger to lightly moisten half of the edge with water. Fold the wrapper in half to enclose the filling. Starting at the bottom of one side, use your fingers to pinch the ends together along the curved edge to seal; if desired, fold a few pleats as you move along the seam. Set aside on the prepared baking sheet seam side up and press gently so that the bottom flattens slightly. Cover with a damp kitchen towel.

Finish the dish. Heat 1 tablespoon of the coconut oil in the reserved skillet over medium-high heat. Arrange half of the dumplings in the pan flat side down, and cook until deep golden brown, 1 to 2 minutes. Remove the pan from the heat. Add 1/2 cup water, then return to the heat. Cover and cook until the dumplings are heated through, the bottoms are crisp, and all the water has evaporated, 4 to 6 minutes, removing the lid for the last 30 seconds of cooking if necessary to let the remaining water evaporate. Transfer the dumplings to a serving platter or divide among six plates. Repeat these steps with the remaining 1 tablespoon coconut oil and dumplings. Serve with the dipping sauce.

Calories: 233.9 kcal

Fat: 7.7 g

Protein: 6.7 g

Carbohydrates: 35.6 g

Sodium: 985.4 mg

vegetable stir-fry with lemongrass

Long stalks of fresh lemongrass are great if you can get them. If you can find only the trimmed bulbs packaged two to three to a container, you should be able to use all of the bulb after peeling away the tough outer layers.

Quinoa takes about 20 minutes to cook. So before you begin the stir-fry, prepare all your ingredients in advance. Stir-fries are best served as soon as possible after cooking, so it's better to cook the quinoa and have it wait for the stir-fry than the other way around.

SERVES 4

2 lemongrass stalks

$1/2$ cup coconut milk

2 tablespoons fresh lime juice

2 teaspoons honey

1 tablespoon virgin coconut oil

$1/3$ cup thinly sliced shallots

$1/2$ teaspoon red chile paste, or to taste

2 cups broccoli florets

8 ounces green beans, trimmed and cut into 2-inch
    pieces (about $2^{1}/2$ cups)

2 carrots, thinly sliced into strips 2 inches long by
    $1/4$ inch wide

2 bell peppers (red, yellow, orange, or a mix), cored,
    seeded, and thinly sliced

Quinoa (page 262), for serving

$1/2$ cup coarsely chopped cashews or Brazil nuts,
    toasted (page 96)

$1/4$ cup torn fresh basil leaves

Peel away the tough outer layers of the lemongrass stalks and use a sharp knife to thinly slice the bottom 4 to 6 inches of the tender bulb. Set aside.

In a 2-cup glass measure or a small bowl, stir together the coconut milk, lime juice, honey, and $1/2$ cup water. Set aside.

Place a large skillet or wok over medium-high heat and heat for about 20 seconds. Add the oil, the reserved lemongrass, and the shallots and cook, stirring, until the shallots are lightly browned, about $1^1/2$ minutes. Stir in the chile paste with 1 to 2 tablespoons of water and cook, stirring, for 1 minute.

Add the broccoli and cook, stirring occasionally, for 1 minute. Stir in the green beans, carrots, and bell peppers. Pour in the coconut milk mixture, cover, and simmer until the vegetables are crisp-tender, 2 to 4 minutes.

Divide the quinoa among four dishes. Spoon the vegetables and sauce over the grain. Sprinkle each serving with the cashews and basil leaves. Serve.

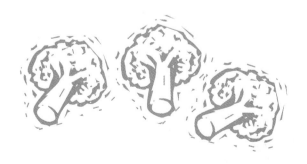

Calories: 423.0 kcal

Fat: 20.3 g

Protein: 12.2 g

Carbohydrates: 54.5 g

Sodium: 79.1 mg

*Nutritional information does not

include quinoa (see page 262).

almond and vegetable pad thai This

recipe comes together easily, especially if you chop all
the vegetables and prepare the almond sauce while the
water for the noodles is coming to a boil. As soon as
you add the noodles to the water, start the stir-fry so
that the vegetables and noodles are ready to be tossed
together at the same time. SERVES 4

1/4 cup plus 2 tablespoons almond butter
1 1/2 tablespoons rice wine vinegar
1 tablespoon fresh lime juice
1 tablespoon honey
1 1/2 teaspoons low-sodium tamari
1 teaspoon red chile paste
1/4 teaspoon toasted sesame oil
8 ounces whole-wheat spaghettini
1 tablespoon virgin coconut oil
1 tablespoon minced garlic
1 tablespoon minced fresh ginger
1/2 cup scallions (white and green parts), cut into
    1-inch pieces before measuring
2 carrots, sliced in thin strips about 2 inches long and
    1/4 inch wide
1 red bell pepper, cored, seeded, and thinly sliced
1 cup shredded fresh spinach

GARNISH
1/2 cup seeded and sliced English cucumber
1/2 cup bean sprouts
1/2 cup fresh cilantro leaves
1/2 cup sliced almonds, toasted (page 96)
Lime wedges

Bring a large pot of water to a boil.

In a blender, place 2 tablespoons water, the almond butter, vinegar, lime juice, honey, tamari, chile paste, and sesame oil. Process until well blended and smooth. Set sauce aside.

When the water comes to a boil, add the noodles and cook until al dente, about 6 minutes, or according to package directions.

While the noodles are cooking, cook the vegetables. In a large skillet or wok, heat the coconut oil over medium-high heat. Add the garlic, ginger, and scallions and cook, stirring, until lightly browned, about 2 minutes. Add the carrots and bell pepper and cook, stirring frequently, until crisp-tender, about 2 minutes. Stir in the spinach and remove the pan from the heat.

When the noodles are done, drain them and transfer them to a large bowl. Add the vegetables and the sauce. Toss to combine.

Divide the noodles among four bowls and garnish each with cucumber, bean sprouts, cilantro, almonds, and a lime wedge. Serve.

Calories: 486.0 kcal

Fat: 22.0 g

Protein: 17.8 g

Carbohydrates: 63.0 g

Sodium: 168.9 mg

*Nutritional information does not include garnishes.

linguine with zucchini, grape tomatoes, and creamy lemon-yogurt sauce SERVES 4

8 ounces whole-wheat linguine
$^1/_2$ cup nonfat plain Greek yogurt
$^1/_4$ cup grated Parmesan cheese
1 teaspoon grated lemon zest
$^1/_4$ teaspoon salt
$^1/_4$ teaspoon ground black pepper
1 tablespoon olive oil
3 medium (8-ounce) zucchini, cut into thin strips
    3 inches long and $^1/_4$ inch wide
2 garlic cloves, thinly sliced
$^1/_2$ pint grape or cherry tomatoes, halved lengthwise

Bring a large pot of water to a boil. Add the linguine and cook about 9 minutes, or according to the package directions. Drain the pasta and reserve $^1/_4$ cup of the cooking water.

Meanwhile, in a large bowl, stir together the yogurt, Parmesan, lemon zest, and salt and pepper. Set aside.

In a large skillet, heat the olive oil over medium-high heat. Add the zucchini and cook just until wilted, about 1 minute. Use a spoon to push the zucchini aside so a space on the bottom of the pan is clear. Add the garlic and cook until fragrant and beginning to brown, about 1 minute. Mix the garlic into the zucchini. Stir in the tomatoes and cook until softened, 1 to 2 minutes.

Calories: 302.7 kcal
Fat: 7.2 g
Protein: 14.4 g
Carbohydrates: 49.0 g
Sodium: 254.7 mg

Transfer the zucchini mixture to the yogurt mixture and stir gently to combine. Add the drained linguine and toss gently to combine. Add the reserved pasta cooking water a tablespoon at a time, if necessary, to thin it. Divide among four bowls and serve.

MASTER YOUR MICROWAVE

There have been many misconceptions over the years about the safety of microwave ovens. At the moment, there is no evidence of any health hazards associated with their use and nothing that would suggest avoiding them. Microwave cooking causes the water molecules in food to vibrate, producing the heat that cooks your food. It doesn't reduce food's nutritional value, and in some cases it's just the opposite. For example, vegetables that are microwaved retain more of their nutrients than vegetables that are steamed.

To be smart, when using your microwave, follow the instruction manual. Don't operate it if the door seems damaged or broken. Never put any kind of metal in the microwave. And don't stand next to the microwave for long periods of time while it's in use.

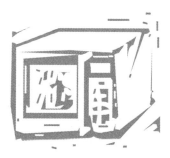

barley risotto with asparagus and lemon

White peppercorns are the same seeds as the more familiar black peppercorns; they are just picked at a different stage of ripeness than the black and treated to remove their outer layer. White pepper is nice in recipes such as this one because it doesn't add unsightly black flecks. The heat of white pepper can be a little more intense than that of black, so use it sparingly and taste as you go. SERVES 4

1 pound asparagus

1 tablespoon olive oil

2 cups thinly sliced leeks (white and green parts)

1 cup pearled barley

1/2 cup dry white wine

1/2 teaspoon salt

3 tablespoons plus 4 teaspoons grated Parmesan
    cheese

1 teaspoon grated lemon zest

1 teaspoon fresh lemon juice, or to taste

1/4 cup thinly sliced fresh mint leaves

1/8 teaspoon freshly ground white or black pepper, or
    to taste

Prepare a bowl of ice water. Trim and discard the stems of the asparagus (or save those ends for veggie broth, page 264). Cut the asparagus into 1-inch lengths. Set the tips aside.

Place the sliced stems into a microwave-safe bowl with a cover. Microwave on high until the asparagus is bright green and just tender, about 2 minutes. Immediately plunge the asparagus into the ice water to stop the cooking. When cool, drain and set aside with the tips.

In a large saucepan, heat the olive oil over medium heat. Add the leeks and cook, stirring occasionally, until softened, about 3 minutes. Add the barley and stir to coat with oil. Cook, stirring occasionally, for 2 minutes. Stir in the wine and cook until it is absorbed.

Stir in 2 cups of water and bring to a simmer. Cover and simmer very gently until the water is absorbed and the barley is tender, 35 to 45 minutes; if the water is absorbed but the barley is not yet tender, stir in up to 1 cup water, cover, and cook until absorbed.

Stir in the reserved asparagus and the salt. For the next 5 to 10 minutes, gradually stir in 1 cup of water. The barley should be creamy and tender to the bite. Remove the pan from the heat and stir in the 3 tablespoons Parmesan, the lemon zest, lemon juice, mint leaves, and pepper. Taste and add more lemon juice and pepper to taste.

Divide the barley among four bowls. Sprinkle 1 teaspoon Parmesan over each bowl, and serve.

Calories: 314.5 kcal
Fat: 7.4 g
Protein: 9.2 g
Carbohydrates: 48.8 g
Sodium: 369.0 mg

winter vegetable couscous Cold

weather is no match for this fragrant stew of

cauliflower, squash, chickpeas, and warm spices. Try

to get your hands on a tube, can, or jar of harissa to

serve with the dish. Harissa is a North African hot

sauce made from chiles and garlic. It adds welcome

heat and bright color to this dish, and it can be found

in the ethnic food sections of many grocery stores or in

Middle Eastern markets. SERVES 8

1 tablespoon olive oil
1 medium red onion, coarsely chopped
1 tablespoon chopped garlic
2 teaspoons ground coriander
1 teaspoon ground cumin
$1/2$ teaspoon turmeric
$1/2$ teaspoon ground cinnamon
$1/8$ teaspoon ground cloves
$1/2$ teaspoon salt
$1/4$ teaspoon ground black pepper
1 medium head cauliflower (about 2 pounds), separated
    into florets
1 medium butternut squash or small pumpkin (about
    3 pounds), peeled, seeded, and cut into 1-inch pieces
2 teaspoons honey
1 (15-ounce) can no- or low-sodium chickpeas, rinsed
    and drained
4 cups cooked Whole-Wheat Couscous (from about
    $1^1/3$ cups dried; page 261)
$1/2$ cup sliced almonds, toasted (page 96)
Harissa, for serving (optional)

In a Dutch oven or other large, heavy pot, heat the olive oil over medium heat. Add the onion and cook, stirring occasionally, until softened, about 4 minutes. Stir in the garlic and cook until fragrant, about 1 minute. Stir in the coriander, cumin, turmeric, cinnamon, cloves, and salt and pepper and cook for 1 minute. Add the cauliflower and squash, and stir to coat with the spices. Add 3 cups water and the honey. Bring to a boil over high heat, cover, reduce the heat, and simmer until the vegetables are somewhat soft, about 5 minutes. Stir in the chickpeas. Simmer, covered, until the vegetables are fork-tender but not mushy, stirring once or twice, 5 to 8 minutes. All the vegetables should be tender enough to cut with the side of a fork, but still hold their shapes.

To serve, spread the couscous over a large serving platter, and using a slotted spoon, mound the vegetables in the center. Pour some of the broth over the vegetables and sprinkle with the almonds. Pass the remaining broth and the harissa, if using, while sitting at the table.

Calories: 305.4 kcal
Fat: 6.1 g
Protein: 11.4 g
Carbohydrates: 56.5 g
Sodium: 151.8 mg

quinoa-stuffed peppers SERVES 4

3/4 cup quinoa

4 large red or yellow bell peppers

1 tablespoon olive oil

1 red onion, chopped

3 ounces cremini or button mushrooms, sliced (about
    1 cup)

2 garlic cloves, chopped

1/4 teaspoon crushed red pepper flakes (optional)

1 tablespoon tomato paste

1 medium zucchini, halved lengthwise and thinly sliced
    crosswise

1 (14-ounce) can diced tomatoes, drained

1 tablespoon chopped fresh oregano leaves, or
    1 teaspoon dried

1/4 teaspoon salt

1/4 teaspoon pepper

2 cups Simple Marinara Sauce (page 266), for serving

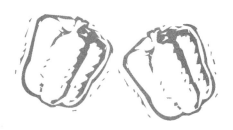

In a small saucepan, bring $1^{1}/2$ cups water to a boil. Place the quinoa in a strainer and rinse under cold running water until the water runs clear. Stir the quinoa into the boiling water, cover, and simmer until the quinoa is tender and the water is absorbed, about 15 minutes. Let stand, covered, for 5 minutes. Fluff with a fork and set aside.

Meanwhile, use a sharp paring knife to cut out the core from the peppers. Pull out any seeds and rinse the peppers inside and out. Place them cut side down on a microwave-safe plate. Microwave on high power until slightly softened, 3 to 4 minutes. Set aside to cool.

In a large skillet, heat the olive oil over medium heat. Add the onion, mushrooms, garlic, and red pepper flakes, if using. Continue to cook, stirring occasionally, until the mushrooms are golden brown, about 8 minutes.

Stir in the tomato paste and cook for 1 minute. Stir in the zucchini, tomatoes, oregano, and salt and pepper and cook for about 2 minutes. Stir in the quinoa and remove the pan from the heat.

Place the peppers cut side up in a medium roasting pan. Spoon the filling into the peppers and fill the pan with water $1/2$ inch deep. Bake until the peppers are tender and the top of the filling is lightly browned and crunchy, about 30 minutes.

Meanwhile, in a small saucepan, heat the marinara over low heat. When the peppers are cooked, place one on each of four plates. Spoon the sauce alongside or on top and serve.

Calories: 297.9 kcal

Fat: 7.9 g

Protein: 9.7 g

Carbohydrates: 49.1 g

Sodium: 563.9 mg

*Nutritional analysis includes marinara.

black bean chili

Chipotles in adobo are smoked jalapeño peppers packed in a tangy tomato sauce. They add fabulous smoky flavor and heat to any dish. You won't need many, so buy them whole packed in a small can and chop up just what you need for this recipe. The rest are easily frozen: place one chile and a spoonful of sauce in each cube of an ice cube tray. You may leave them there until needed or transfer them all to a freezer-safe container and pull out or chop off what you need. SERVES 8

2 cups dried black beans
2 tablespoons olive oil
2 medium onions, finely chopped
2 green bell peppers, cored, seeded, and finely chopped
6 garlic cloves, finely chopped
1 tablespoon chili powder
1 tablespoon ground cumin
1 tablespoon dried oregano
1/2 teaspoon ground cinnamon
1/4 teaspoon ground black pepper
1 (28-ounce) can diced tomatoes with their juice
1 teaspoon grated orange zest
1 cup fresh orange juice
1 tablespoon honey
1 to 3 teaspoons chopped chipotle chiles in adobo
    (optional)
1/2 cup medium-grind bulgur
1/2 teaspoon salt

^{1}/2 cup nonfat plain Greek yogurt
3 tablespoons minced scallions (white and green parts)
3 tablespoons minced fresh cilantro
8 lime wedges

Place the beans in a colander and pick them over to remove any debris, then rinse and drain. Place them in a Dutch oven or other large, heavy pot and add water to cover by 2 inches. Bring to a boil. Reduce the heat to low and simmer, partially covered, until almost tender, about 1 hour. Drain and set aside.

Heat the oil in the same large pot over medium-high heat until hot but not smoking. Add the onions and bell peppers and cook, stirring occasionally, until just starting to brown, 8 to 10 minutes. Stir in the garlic and cook until fragrant, about 30 seconds. Stir in the chili powder, cumin, oregano, cinnamon, and black pepper. Then stir in the tomatoes, orange zest and juice, honey, chipotle, and 3 cups water. Add the reserved beans. Return to a simmer and cook, partially covered, checking occasionally and adding more water as needed, until the beans are just tender to the bite, about 1^1/2 hours. Stir in the bulgur 15 minutes before removing the chili from the heat. Taste and add up to ^{1}/2 teaspoon salt for flavor.

Divide the chili into eight bowls and top each serving with the yogurt, scallions, cilantro, and a lime wedge, if desired, or pass the toppings separately at the table.

Calories: 297.2 kcal

Fat: 4.7 g

Protein: 14.6 g

Carbohydrates: 52.9 g

Sodium: 414.4 mg

*Nutritional analysis does not include garnishes.

baked ratatouille with parmesan

SERVES 6

2 tablespoons olive oil

1 medium eggplant (about 3/4 pound), cut into
   1/2-inch cubes

1/2 teaspoon salt

1 medium red onion, diced

1 tablespoon finely chopped garlic

1/4 teaspoon crushed red pepper flakes

1 tablespoon tomato paste

2 red bell peppers, cut into 1/2-inch cubes

1 (28-ounce) can diced tomatoes, drained

1 medium zucchini (about 6 ounces), cut into
   1/4-inch-thick half-moons

1 medium summer squash (about 6 ounces), cut into
   1/4-inch-thick half-moons

2 (15-ounce) cans no-sodium chickpeas, rinsed and
   drained

1 tablespoon chopped fresh thyme leaves, or
   1 teaspoon dried

1 tablespoon chopped fresh marjoram leaves, or
   1 teaspoon dried

1/4 teaspoon ground black pepper

2 tablespoons grated Parmesan cheese

Preheat the oven to 400°F. Have ready a 3-quart baking dish.

In a skillet over medium-high heat, heat 1 tablespoon of the olive oil until hot but not smoking. Add the eggplant and a pinch of the salt. Cook, stirring occasionally, until lightly browned, about 8 minutes. Spread the eggplant in the bottom of the baking dish.

Wipe the skillet clean and heat the remaining 1 tablespoon olive oil over medium-low heat. Add the onion, garlic, and red pepper flakes and cook, stirring occasionally, until softened, about 4 minutes. Stir in the tomato paste and cook for about 1 minute more. Add the peppers and cook until softened, about 8 minutes.

Stir in the drained tomatoes, the zucchini, summer squash, chickpeas, thyme, marjoram, remaining salt, and pepper. Bring to a boil, cover, and simmer for 5 minutes.

Spoon the mixture evenly over the eggplant. Sprinkle the cheese evenly over the top. Bake until bubbling and lightly browned on top, about 30 minutes. Let stand for 10 minutes before serving.

Calories: 269.6 kcal
Fat: 7.0 g
Protein: 11.5 g
Carbohydrates: 40.2 g
Sodium: 568.0 mg

side dishes

COCONUT-GINGER YELLOW RICE

COUSCOUS WITH CARROTS, PARSNIPS, AND ORANGE

BLACK BEANS AND RICE

BARLEY WITH ROASTED CAULIFLOWER AND ALMONDS

RUSSET POTATO SALAD WITH ARUGULA AND LEMON

CREAMY CUCUMBER AND YOGURT SALAD

ROASTED SHIITAKES WITH FRESH THYME

SAUTÉED ARAME AND CARROTS

NO-CREAM CREAMED SPINACH

ROASTED GARLIC BEETS

BRAISED BABY ARTICHOKES WITH TOMATOES

SMASHED SWEET POTATOES WITH COCONUT MILK

THAI SPAGHETTI SQUASH

coconut-ginger yellow rice SERVES 4

1 teaspoon virgin coconut oil
1 shallot, chopped
1 teaspoon turmeric
$1/4$ teaspoon salt
$1/4$ teaspoon ground black pepper
$3/4$ cup coconut milk
Thin quarter-size slice of fresh ginger
1 cup long-grain brown rice
4 lime wedges, for garnish

In a medium saucepan, heat the oil over low heat. Add the shallot, turmeric, and salt and pepper. Cook, stirring occasionally, until the shallot begins to soften, 1 to 2 minutes.

Stir in the coconut milk, ginger, and $1^1/4$ cups water. Increase the heat to medium and bring to a boil. Stir in the rice and return to a boil. Reduce the heat, cover, and simmer gently until the rice is tender and the liquid is absorbed, 45 to 50 minutes. Remove the pan from the heat and let stand, covered, for 5 minutes. Remove and discard the ginger and fluff with a fork just before serving. Garnish with lime wedges, if desired.

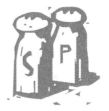

Calories: 276.5 kcal
Fat: 11.6 g
Protein: 5.0 g
Carbohydrates: 39.9 g
Sodium: 134.2 mg

couscous with carrots, parsnips, and orange

Inspired by rice pilaf, which is delicious but takes a while to prepare, this flavorful side dish comes together in minutes. SERVES 6

1 tablespoon olive oil
$1/2$ cup finely chopped red onion
1 medium carrot, sliced (about $1/2$ cup)
1 small parsnip, sliced (about $1/2$ cup)
$1/2$ teaspoon ground cumin
$1/8$ teaspoon smoked paprika
Juice of 1 orange
1 teaspoon grated orange zest
1 cup whole-wheat couscous
$1/4$ teaspoon salt
$1/8$ teaspoon ground black pepper
2 tablespoons slivered almonds, toasted (page 96; optional)

In a small saucepan, heat the olive oil over medium heat. Add the onion, carrot, and parsnip. Cook, stirring occasionally, until softened, about 8 minutes. Stir in the cumin and paprika, and cook for 1 minute.

Meanwhile, pour the orange juice into a measuring cup. Add enough water to make $1^1/4$ cups. Pour the juice and water into the saucepan. Bring to a boil. Reduce the heat and simmer, partially covered, for 2 minutes. Stir in the orange zest, couscous, and salt and pepper. Cover and simmer for 2 minutes. Stir, cover, and remove the pan from the heat. Let stand for 5 minutes. Fluff with a fork. Sprinkle with almonds before serving, if you like.

Calories: 116.1 kcal
Fat: 2.8 g
Protein: 3.2 g
Carbohydrates: 20.8 g
Sodium: 89.0 mg

black beans and rice SERVES 8 TO 10

1 cup dried black beans, picked over and rinsed
1 tablespoon olive oil
1 cup chopped red onion
2 garlic cloves, finely chopped
1 tablespoon tomato paste
1 $1/2$ teaspoons ground cumin
1 cup long-grain brown rice
1 (14-ounce) can low-sodium diced tomatoes
$1^1/2$ teaspoons dried oregano
1 fresh or dried bay leaf
$1/2$ teaspoon salt
$1/4$ teaspoon ground black pepper
$1/2$ cup parsley leaves, chopped
$1/2$ teaspoon hot pepper sauce (optional)

In a large saucepan, place the beans and add water to cover by 2 inches. Bring to a boil. Reduce the heat to low and simmer, partially covered, until almost tender, about 1 hour. Drain; set aside.

In the saucepan, heat the olive oil over medium-low heat. Add the onion and garlic and cook until lightly browned, 8 to 10 minutes. Turn the heat to medium and stir in the tomato paste; cook for 1 minute. Stir in the cumin and cook for 1 minute.

Add the rice and cook, stirring, until well incorporated and toasted, about 2 minutes. Stir in 2 cups water, the tomatoes, beans, oregano, bay leaf, and salt and pepper. Bring to a boil. Reduce the heat and simmer, covered, until the liquid is absorbed and the rice and beans are tender to the bite, about 1 hour. Let stand, covered, for 5 minutes.

Add the parsley and the hot sauce, if using, and use a fork to fluff the rice and beans and incorporate the parsley. Remove and discard the bay leaf. Serve.

Calories: 202.4 kcal
Fat: 2.9 g
Protein: 8.0 g
Carbohydrates: 37.0 g
Sodium: 163.9 mg

barley with roasted cauliflower and almonds SERVES 8

1 cup pearled barley
1/2 teaspoon salt
1 small head cauliflower, cut into florets
1 small shallot, thinly sliced
1/4 cup sliced almonds
1 tablespoon olive oil
1 teaspoon honey
1/8 teaspoon ground black pepper
1/4 cup fresh parsley leaves, chopped

Preheat the oven to 425°F.

In a medium saucepan, place the barley, 1/4 teaspoon of the salt, and 3 cups water. Bring to a boil. Reduce the heat to low, cover, and simmer until the barley is tender, 30 to 40 minutes. Let stand, covered, for 5 minutes.

Meanwhile, in a medium bowl, place the cauliflower florets, shallot, almonds, olive oil, honey, remaining 1/4 teaspoon salt, and the pepper. Mix well until the cauliflower is well coated with olive oil and honey. Transfer to a shallow roasting pan and spread the mixture in a single layer. Bake until the cauliflower is tender and brown in spots, about 20 minutes, stirring occasionally.

Transfer the cauliflower to the saucepan with the barley. Add the parsley and use a fork to mix them. Serve.

Calories: 137.0 kcal
Fat: 3.8 g
Protein: 3.9 g
Carbohydrates: 23.1 g
Sodium: 133.3 mg

MASTERING ALLERGIES

Recent studies have shown that the B vitamin folate may help keep allergic reactions in check. With both asthma and allergies, the immune system has an exaggerated response to foreign substances such as dust and pollen, which triggers respiratory troubles. Folic acid has been shown to dampen that response and to dampen inflammation at the core of these conditions. *Eat:* asparagus, broccoli, oranges, kidney beans, collard greens, black-eyed peas, spinach, lentils, and avocado.

Check out my Vegetable Stir-Fry with Lemongrass (page 190), and Barley Risotto with Asparagus and Lemon (page 196).

russet potato salad with arugula and lemon

Cook the potatoes until they are just tender or they will fall apart when mixed with the other ingredients. The resistant starch in russet potatoes is more bioavailable if they are cold, but they must be warm to properly absorb the tasty vinaigrette, so be sure to pour it over just after they're cooked. SERVES 10

2 ounces arugula leaves, stems trimmed, leaves coarsely chopped (about 2 cups)
3 pounds russet potatoes, scrubbed and cut into 3/4-inch pieces
1 large head garlic, cloves separated and chopped
3/4 teaspoon salt
Grated zest and juice of 1 lemon
About 2 tablespoons champagne vinegar
1 teaspoon Dijon mustard
Freshly ground pepper to taste
$^1/_3$ cup extra-virgin olive oil
1 cup chopped celery
3 tablespoons chopped fresh chives or scallion greens

Place the arugula in a large mixing bowl.

In a large saucepan, place the potatoes, garlic, and $^1/_4$ teaspoon of the salt, and add cold water to cover. Bring to a boil. Reduce the heat and simmer, partially covered, until the potatoes are just tender, about 5 minutes. Drain well and transfer to the bowl with the arugula.

Meanwhile, pour the lemon juice into a glass measuring cup. Add enough vinegar to make $^1/_4$ cup. Pour into a small mixing bowl. Add the mustard, grated lemon zest, remaining $^1/_2$ teaspoon salt, and $^1/_4$ teaspoon pepper. Whisk to combine. Whisking constantly, pour in the olive oil in a steady stream.

Pour the vinaigrette over the potatoes and toss gently. Set aside to cool for 30 to 60 minutes, and then refrigerate until cold.

Stir in the celery and chives. Taste for seasoning and add more lemon juice or pepper, if desired. Serve.

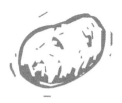

Calories: 187.8 kcal
Fat: 7.7 g
Protein: 3.5 g
Carbohydrates: 27.5 g
Sodium: 127.2 mg

creamy cucumber and yogurt salad

This refreshing salad is delicious with the Mediterranean Lamb Burgers (page 132) and the Grilled Lamb Skewers with Plums (page 130). SERVES 4

1 English cucumber
1 cup nonfat plain Greek yogurt
$1/3$ cup minced red onion
2 tablespoons finely minced fresh mint leaves
1 teaspoon grated lemon zest
1 teaspoon fresh lemon juice, or to taste
$1/8$ teaspoon salt

In a food processor fitted with the shredding attachment or on the coarse side of a box grater, grate the cucumber. Transfer it to a medium bowl and add the yogurt, onion, mint, lemon zest and juice, and the salt. Stir to combine. Serve.

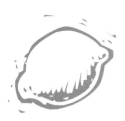

Calories: 41.3 kcal
Fat: 0.0 g
Protein: 4.7 g
Carbohydrates: 5.8 g
Sodium: 77.6 mg

roasted shiitakes with fresh thyme

SERVES 4

1 pound shiitake mushrooms, stems removed, halved if large
1 tablespoon olive oil
4 sprigs fresh thyme
$1/4$ teaspoon salt
$1/4$ teaspoon ground black pepper
Fresh lemon juice to taste (optional)

Preheat the oven to 450°F.

On a large, rimmed baking sheet, arrange the mushrooms. Drizzle with the olive oil and add the thyme sprigs, salt, and pepper. Toss to coat.

Roast the mushrooms, stirring occasionally, until tender and browned, about 20 minutes. Remove and discard the thyme sprigs and add a squeeze of lemon juice, if desired. Serve.

Calories: 79.5 kcal
Fat: 3.7 g
Protein: 1.3 g
Carbohydrates: 12.3 g
Sodium: 123.5 mg

SIMPLE COOKED VEGETABLES

You can enjoy cooked vegetables in dozens of ways following the recipes in this book. And while most of the recipes here are really straightforward, sometimes you just need to throw something together, right? The quickest way I know is to use the microwave, but the most succulent method is roasting—so here's how to do both. Figure about 1 pound of trimmed vegetables will serve 4 people, but you can certainly eat more!

Microwave-Steamed Vegetables

This is my favorite method for quickly cooking fresh green beans, asparagus pieces, broccoli and cauliflower florets, thinly sliced carrots, and cubed russet or sweet potatoes. Place 1 pound of the prepared vegetable in a microwave-safe bowl with a lid. Cover and cook in the microwave on high power until the vegetable is brightly colored and crisp-tender:

- 2 to 3 minutes for asparagus
- 3 to 4 minutes for green beans and thinly sliced carrots
- 3 to 5 minutes for potatoes, less if you want them to say in pieces, more if you're mashing them
- 4 to 5 minutes for broccoli and cauliflower

To enhance their flavor, and better absorb some of their nutrients, after cooking, toss the vegetables with 1 tablespoon extra-virgin olive oil, a pinch of salt, and a bit of freshly ground black pepper.

Roasted Vegetables

Roasting brings out the natural sweetness in vegetables—making them something like vegetable candy—and can be done with very little oil. Use this method for cauliflower, asparagus, turnips, eggplant, carrots, parsnips, russet potatoes, sweet potatoes, bell peppers, zucchini, onions, shallots, or garlic. Roast just one type or mix two or three together in the same pan—make sure all the vegetables are cut to the same size.

I rarely roast any vegetable without throwing a handful of garlic cloves in the pan—usually with their peels still on (that way anyone less enthusiastic about the garlic can easily avoid it).

Most vegetables will take somewhere between 25 and 50 minutes to roast, although asparagus will take considerably less—8 to 12 minutes.

Preheat the oven to 400° F. Spray a large, rimmed baking sheet or jelly-roll pan with olive oil or brush the pan lightly with olive oil.

Cut the cauliflower into florets. Trim the asparagus, the turnips, and the eggplant. Peel and trim the carrots and the parsnips. Scrub the potatoes. Core and remove the seeds from the bell peppers. Peel and trim the onions and the shallots.

Cut the vegetables into uniform pieces—$3/4$ to 1 inch usually works pretty well, although I usually cut peppers and onions into 8 wedges. Shallots can be left whole if they're small.

Place the vegetables on the roasting pan and drizzle over them 2 teaspoons of olive oil. Add a pinch of salt and several grinds of black pepper. Throw in a couple of sprigs of thyme or 1 teaspoon dried rosemary, if desired. Toss to coat. Spread the vegetables in a single layer. Roast until tender and browned, turning the vegetables once or twice during roasting:

- Asparagus: 8 to 12 minutes
- Eggplant, bell peppers, russet potatoes, zucchini, garlic, and shallots: 35 to 40 minutes
- Cauliflower, turnips, carrots, parsnips, sweet potatoes, and onions: 50 to 60 minutes

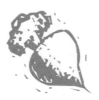

sautéed arame and carrots Dried seaweed is a fabulous addition to your pantry. It keeps for months and can be whipped up in moments to accompany any fish or shellfish recipe. It's especially good with Bay Scallops with Toasted Sesame Seeds (page 168). SERVES 8

2 ounces dried arame (or other shredded seaweed)
1 tablespoon virgin coconut oil
$^1/_2$ cup sliced scallions (white and green parts)
2 large carrots, peeled and cut into 2-inch matchsticks
2 tablespoons minced fresh ginger
$^1/_4$ teaspoon crushed red pepper flakes
3 tablespoons fresh orange juice
1 tablespoon low-sodium tamari
1 teaspoon toasted sesame oil
$^1/_4$ cup fresh cilantro leaves, chopped
1 tablespoon sesame seeds, toasted (page 96)

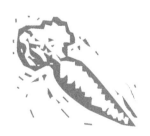

Place the arame in a medium bowl and cover with cold water. Soak for 5 minutes, and drain.

In a heavy skillet, heat the oil over medium heat. Add the scallions, carrots, ginger, and red pepper flakes, and cook, stirring, until the carrots are crisp-tender and the ginger is golden brown, 3 to 5 minutes.

Stir in the arame and cook for 1 minute. Add $^1/2$ cup of water. Cover, raise the heat to medium high, and bring to a boil. Lower the heat and simmer, covered, for about 8 minutes. Remove the cover and cook until most of the liquid has evaporated, 6 to 8 minutes. Stir in the orange juice, tamari, and sesame oil. Cook for 5 minutes.

Remove from the heat and stir in the cilantro. Sprinkle with the sesame seeds and serve.

Calories: 63.4 kcal
Fat: 3.0 g
Protein: 1.5 g
Carbohydrates: 8.4 g
Sodium: 175.4 mg

no-cream creamed spinach

SERVES 4 TO 6

2 pounds fresh spinach (2 to 3 bunches), trimmed,
  washed, and chopped
2 tablespoons olive oil
3/4 cup chopped red onion
2 garlic cloves, finely chopped
1/4 teaspoon salt
2 tablespoons white whole-wheat flour
1 cup almond milk
1 tablespoon fresh lemon juice, or to taste
2 tablespoons sliced almonds, toasted (page 96;
  optional)

In a large skillet, place half of the spinach with the rinse water still clinging to its leaves (or, if the leaves are quite dry, add 1 tablespoon water to the pan). Cover and cook over medium heat until very wilted and tender, about 5 minutes. Transfer the spinach to the work bowl of a food processor or blender and process until smooth.

Wipe the skillet clean, pour in the olive oil, and warm over medium-low heat. Add the onion, garlic, and salt, and cook, stirring occasionally, until softened, about 6 minutes.

Add the flour and cook, stirring occasionally, until toasted and fragrant, about 5 minutes. Stir in the almond milk. Cook until thickened, about 1 minute. Stir in the puréed spinach and transfer the mixture to a bowl.

Calories: 147.4 kcal
Fat: 8.3 g
Protein: 6.4 g
Carbohydrates: 15.2 g
Sodium: 281.9 mg

Add the remaining spinach to the skillet; add 1 tablespoon water to the pan if the leaves are very dry. Cover and cook over medium-high heat until wilted, 3 to 4 minutes, stirring occasionally. Gently fold the puréed spinach and the lemon juice into the wilted spinach. Sprinkle with the almonds, if desired. Serve.

Anti-Cancer Heart Healthy Boosts Metabolism Improves Digestion Boosts Immunity

roasted garlic beets SERVES 4

6 beets, trimmed and scrubbed, halved if very large
4 garlic cloves, unpeeled
3 teaspoons olive oil
1 tablespoon snipped fresh chives
1/4 teaspoon salt
1/4 teaspoon ground black pepper

Preheat the oven to 425°F.

Place the beets and garlic in a small roasting pan. Pour 1 teaspoon of the olive oil over the veggies and stir to coat. Cover the pan with aluminum foil and bake until the beets are tender when pierced with a sharp, thin-bladed knife, about 45 minutes.

Let stand just until cool enough to handle, 5 to 10 minutes. Using a paring knife and your fingers, peel the beets and cut them into bite-size pieces. Place them in a bowl.

Peel the garlic, chop it, and add it to the bowl with the beets. Add the remaining 2 teaspoons olive oil, the chives, and the salt and pepper. Stir to combine. Serve.

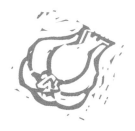

Calories: 59.0 kcal
Fat: 2.5 g
Protein: 1.5 g
Carbohydrates: 8.6 g
Sodium: 178.3 mg

braised baby artichokes with tomatoes SERVES 4

1 lemon, halved, plus 2 tablespoons fresh lemon juice
16 baby artichokes
1 ^{1}/$_2$ tablespoons olive oil
2 ounces shallots, thinly sliced (about ^{1}/$_3$ cup)
4 garlic cloves, finely chopped
6 fresh or canned low-sodium plum tomatoes, chopped
^{1}/$_4$ cup white wine or low-sodium chicken broth or
    Vegetable Broth (page 264), plus more if needed
^{1}/$_4$ teaspoon salt
^{1}/$_4$ teaspoon ground black pepper
1 tablespoon chopped fresh flat-leaf parsley

Fill a large bowl with cold water and squeeze into it the juice from the halved lemon; drop the halves into the water. This lemon water will keep the trimmed artichokes from browning. Pull off the tough outer leaves from the artichokes. Cut off the top ^{1}/$_2$ inch and slice off the stems. Halve the artichokes through the stems and place them in the bowl of water.

In a large skillet, heat the olive oil over medium heat. Add the shallots and garlic, and cook until softened, stirring occasionally, about 2 minutes. Drain the artichokes and add them to the pan. Stir and cook until they begin to brown at the edges, about 5 minutes. Add the tomatoes, wine, lemon juice, and salt and pepper. Cover and simmer until the artichokes are tender, about 15 minutes, adding a little water or broth if the pan starts to look very dry.

Stir in the parsley and serve.

Calories: 155.5 kcal
Fat: 6.2 g
Protein: 6.0 g
Carbohydrates: 22.7 g
Sodium: 297.3 mg

smashed sweet potatoes with coconut milk
Leaving the peels on the potatoes preserves vital nutrients and adds really nice texture. Who says potatoes can't be a health food—and a delicious one at that? SERVES 4

1^{1}/$_{2}$ pounds sweet potatoes, scrubbed and cut into ^{3}/$_{4}$-inch chunks
^{1}/$_{2}$ cup coconut milk
^{1}/$_{4}$ teaspoon salt
Pinch of grated nutmeg

Place the sweet potatoes in a glass microwave-safe bowl. Cover and microwave on high until very tender, 4 to 5 minutes.

Transfer the hot, cooked potatoes to a mixing bowl. Add the coconut milk, salt, and nutmeg. Use a potato masher to mash the potatoes and combine with the other ingredients. Serve.

Calories: 161.3 kcal
Fat: 6.1 g
Protein: 2.5 g
Carbohydrates: 25.5 g
Sodium: 191.0 mg

thai spaghetti squash SERVES 4

1 (2-pound) spaghetti squash
1 teaspoon virgin coconut oil
1 small shallot, thinly sliced
1/4 teaspoon red curry paste
1/3 cup coconut milk
2 tablespoons chopped fresh cilantro leaves

With a sharp, thin-bladed knife, pierce the squash in four or five places around its perimeter; be sure to pierce far enough to reach the center of the squash. Place in the microwave and cook on high power until tender when pushed with your fingers, 15 to 20 minutes; turn the squash every few minutes if the microwave does not have a turntable. Let stand for 10 minutes.

Cut the squash in half through the stem and remove the seeds. Scrape the flesh off the skin into a bowl, and discard the skin. Use a fork to shred the squash into strands. Set aside.

In a large skillet, heat the oil over medium heat. Add the shallot and cook, stirring occasionally, until softened, about 3 minutes. Add the curry paste and cook for 1 minute. Add the coconut milk, and bring to a simmer. Simmer gently for 1 minute.

Add the squash and use tongs to toss it and coat it thoroughly with the sauce. Cook until warmed through, 1 to 2 minutes. Add the cilantro and toss to mix well. Serve.

Calories: 103.1 kcal
Fat: 5.7 g
Protein: 1.8 g
Carbohydrates: 13.9 g
Sodium: 38.1 mg

snacks

BANANA-ALMOND SMOOTHIE

AÇAI BERRY AND POMEGRANATE SMOOTHIE

PAPAYA AND KIWI SUMMER ROLLS

CHEDDAR AND APPLE SLICES WITH CINNAMON

ROASTED RUSSET FRIES

BAKED GARLIC PITA CHIPS

HUMMUS

GUACAMOLE

TOMATILLO AND TOMATO SALSA

BLACK BEAN DIP

TRAIL MIX

SPICED ROASTED ALMONDS

banana-almond smoothie SERVES 2

1 cup sliced banana (from about 1 large banana)
1 cup almond milk
1 tablespoon almond butter
1 tablespoon ground flaxseed
1 teaspoon vanilla extract
2 cups ice cubes (about 8 cubes)

Calories: 167.6 kcal
Fat: 7.8 g
Protein: 3.2 g
Carbohydrates: 22.6 g
Sodium: 112.6 mg

In a blender, place the banana, almond milk, almond butter, flaxseed, and vanilla. Blend until very well combined, 45 to 60 seconds. Add the ice cubes and blend until smooth. Pour into two glasses and serve.

HEALTH BENEFITS:
Anti-Cancer Heart Healthy Boosts Immunity Boosts Metabolism Healthy Skin Strong Bones Improves Digestion

açai berry and pomegranate smoothie SERVES 4

1 (3^1/2-ounce) packet frozen açai berry puree, partially thawed
1 cup pomegranate juice
1 cup low-fat plain kefir
2 scoops whey protein powder
1 tablespoon agave syrup
2 cups ice cubes (about 8 cubes)

Calories: 157.9 kcal
Fat: 3.2 g
Protein: 15.7 g
Carbohydrates: 21.3 g
Sodium: 76.4 mg

In a blender, place the açai berry puree, pomegranate juice, kefir, whey protein powder, agave syrup, and ice. Cover and blend until smooth.

Divide among four glasses and serve.

MASTER YOUR DRINKING WATER

Should you go bottled or tap? Easy! Tap. Just because water is bottled does not mean that it is contaminant-free. In fact, quite the opposite is true. City water is highly regulated and monitored for safety; bottled water is not. Technically, bottled water is monitored by the FDA, but it turns out that about 70 percent of bottled water sold in a state is exempt from federal regulation. And many bottled waters have tested positive for bacteria, man-made chemicals, and arsenic. Going with tap saves you money and saves the environment by keeping the landfills clean and reducing the carbon emissions caused by transporting the water from exotic locations to your fridge. But wait, you're not out of the woods yet. Drinking tap water still leaves you at risk for lead, chlorine, pesticides, fungicides, herbicides, hormones, antibiotics, and nitrates. You can check the quality of your local water by calling the EPA's safe-water hotline at 1-800-426-4791, or by visiting their Web site, www.epa.gov/safewater. Also check out the national drinking water quality database put together by the Environmental Working Group (www.ewg.org).

Your best bet is to filter your tap water. Reverse osmosis is an option. It removes all heavy metals, viruses, and some pharmaceuticals. Or you can go with an activated carbon filter. The quality varies from product to product, but most will remove heavy metals, pesticides, and some pharmaceuticals.

HEALTH BENEFITS:
Anti-Cancer Boosts Metabolism Healthy Skin Improves Digestion Miscellaneous

papaya and kiwi summer rolls

SERVES 4

3 tablespoons honey
$1/2$ teaspoon grated lime zest
1 tablespoon fresh lime juice
$1/8$ teaspoon chipotle chile powder
4 kiwi fruit, peeled
$1/2$ large papaya, seeded and peeled
$1/3$ cup hazelnuts, coarsely chopped, toasted (page 96)
$1/4$ cup fresh mint leaves, chopped
8 (8-inch) round rice-paper wrappers

MASTERING STRESS

- **For brighter moods:** Stock up on foods with B vitamins, as they stimulate the brain's production of serotonin. *Eat:* almonds, pistachios, salmon, scallops, shrimp, walnuts, and poultry.
- **For managing anger:** Potassium is not only a great natural diuretic, but it also lowers blood pressure and helps keep short tempers in check. *Eat:* avocados, bananas, black beans, potatoes, and white beans.
- **For better sleep:** Magnesium acts as a natural tranquilizer, relaxing muscles, blood vessels, and your gastrointestinal tract. *Eat:* chickpeas, lentils, oatmeal, pumpkin seeds, spinach, and swiss chard.
  Check out Roasted Salmon with Pepita and Cumin Seed Crust (page 150) and Almond-Crusted Chicken Breasts (page 112).

In a small bowl, place the honey, lime zest, lime juice, chile powder, and 1 tablespoon water. Whisk together until well combined. Set aside.

Slice the kiwi lengthwise in half. Cut each half crosswise into thin slices. Set aside on a large platter. Cut the papaya into thin strips about 1/2 inch wide and 3 to 4 inches long. Set aside with the kiwi. Place the hazelnuts and mint on the platter with the fruit.

Prepare a bowl of warm water. Lay a clean kitchen towel on the work surface.

For each roll, soak a rice paper wrapper in the water until it is softened, about 45 seconds. Gently lay the wrapper flat on the towel and pat it dry. In the center of the wrapper, lay one-eighth of each of the sliced kiwi, sliced papaya, hazelnuts, and mint. Pull the top of the wrapper down over the filling. Fold in both sides of the wrapper; the wrapper will stick to itself. Pull the bottom of the wrapper up and over the filling and wrap it snugly around the filling to make a tight cylinder.

Transfer the summer rolls as shaped to a clean serving platter and cover with a damp cloth until ready to serve. Serve with the dipping sauce.

Calories: 235.9 kcal
Fat: 6.7 g
Protein: 3.4 g
Carbohydrates: 44.8 g
Sodium: 31.0 mg

cheddar and apple slices with cinnamon SERVES 1

Calories: 107.6 kcal
Fat: 4.7 g
Protein: 8.3 g
Carbohydrates: 10.7 g
Sodium: 172.8 mg

$^1/_2$ medium apple, cored and cut into 4 wedges
$^1/_8$ teaspoon ground cinnamon
1 ounce low-fat Cheddar cheese, cut into 4 slices

Place the apple on a small serving plate. Sprinkle the wedges with the cinnamon. Top each wedge with a slice of Cheddar. Serve.

roasted russet fries SERVES 8

Calories: 136.8 kcal
Fat: 5.3 g
Protein: 2.4 g
Carbohydrates: 20.5 g
Sodium: 125.7 mg

4 medium-large russet potatoes, scrubbed but not
    peeled
3 tablespoons extra-virgin olive oil
$^1/_2$ teaspoon salt
$^1/_2$ teaspoon pepper
Ketchup (page 268), for serving

Preheat the oven to 475°F. Have ready two rimmed baking sheets.

Cut 1 potato lengthwise into quarters. Cut each quarter lengthwise into 2 to 3 wedges. Repeat with the remaining potatoes. Place the potatoes in a large mixing bowl. Add the olive oil, salt, and pepper. Toss gently to thoroughly coat the potatoes.

Arrange the wedges in a single layer on the baking sheet. Bake until the potatoes are crispy and brown, 35 to 40 minutes. Serve warm with Ketchup.

baked garlic pita chips

Store-bought pita chips are usually jam-packed with sodium, and that's often the least of the garbage in those bags. Making them at home is a snap. Whip up a batch when you have a few minutes and they'll keep for days. They are heavenly with any one of the dips and spreads on the pages that follow—so you'll never be tempted to reach for that bagged junk. MAKES 48 CHIPS; 16 SERVINGS

Olive oil spray for the baking sheets
4 (6-inch) whole-wheat pita breads
3 tablespoons extra-virgin olive oil
1 garlic clove, crushed
1/4 teaspoon salt

Preheat the oven to 400°F. Spray two rimmed baking sheets with olive oil.

Working with one pita at a time, use a pair of kitchen scissors to cut along the outside edges and separate each into 2 circles. Stack the circles and cut them in half. Cut each half into 3 wedges; you'll have 48 triangles. Arrange the triangles on the prepared baking sheets so that the side that was the inside of the pita is facing up.

In a small dish, combine the olive oil with the garlic. Lightly brush each pita triangle with the oil and garlic mixture; brush only the side that is facing up. Sprinkle the pitas with the salt.

Bake until the chips are lightly browned around the edges and crisp, turning the pans once during baking, 8 to 10 minutes. Let cool slightly or completely before serving. (Pita chips can be stored in an airtight container for 3 to 4 days.)

Calories 53.6 kcal
Fat: 2.9 g
Protein: 1.1 g
Carbohydrates: 6.2 g
Sodium: 89.9 mg

hummus
Ground sumac adds a welcome tanginess; see Resources (page 270) for notes on where to find it. MAKES 2 CUPS; 16 (2-TABLESPOON) SERVINGS

1 (15-ounce) can no-sodium chickpeas
1/4 cup fresh lemon juice, or to taste
3 tablespoons tahini
2 garlic cloves, finely chopped
1/2 teaspoon salt
2 teaspoons extra-virgin olive oil, for garnish
1/8 teaspoon sumac or sweet, hot, or smoked paprika, for garnish
Baked Garlic Pita Chips (page 231), for serving

Place a strainer over a bowl and drain the chickpeas; reserve 1/4 cup of the captured liquid.

In the work bowl of a food processor, place the lemon juice, tahini, garlic, and salt. Process until combined. Add the drained chickpeas and the reserved liquid. Process until very smooth, scraping down the sides of the work bowl once or twice or as needed. Taste and add more lemon juice if desired. (The hummus can be stored in a tightly sealed container in the refrigerator for up to 1 week.)

For a single snack, place 2 tablespoons of the hummus in a small bowl. Drizzle with 1/8 teaspoon olive oil and sprinkle a pinch of sumac over it. Serve with 3 pita chips.

To serve a crowd, transfer the hummus to a small serving bowl. If desired, use the back of a spoon to make a shallow well in the surface of the hummus; pour in the olive oil. Sprinkle the top with the sumac. Serve with the pita chips.

Calories: 49.4 kcal
Fat: 2.1 g
Protein: 2.0 g
Carbohydrates: 5.9 g
Sodium: 68.3 mg

Anti-Cancer Boosts Metabolism Healthy Skin Improves Digestion Miscellaneous

guacamole MAKES 2 CUPS; 16 (2-TABLESPOON) SERVINGS

2 plum tomatoes, finely chopped (about 1 cup)

$1/4$ cup finely chopped red onion

2 tablespoons fresh lime juice

2 tablespoons chopped fresh cilantro leaves

$1/2$ teaspoon seeded and minced fresh chiles

$1/4$ teaspoon salt

$1/4$ teaspoon ground cumin

2 small, ripe avocados, pitted and peeled

In a medium bowl, gently combine the tomatoes, onion, lime juice, cilantro, chiles, salt, and cumin. Stir. Add the avocados and use a fork to gently mash and combine them with the other ingredients.

(Guacamole is best served soon after preparation, but it can be stored in a tightly covered container in the refrigerator for up to 2 days.)

Calories: 43.3 kcal

Fat: 3.7 g

Protein: 0.6 g

Carbohydrates: 2.9 g

Sodium: 32.4 mg

tomatillo and tomato salsa

MAKES 2^1/$_2$ CUPS; 16 (2^1/$_2$-TABLESPOON) SERVINGS

^{1}/$_2$ pound tomatillos (about 6), papery husks removed,
   tomatillos rinsed and diced
^{1}/$_2$ pound ripe, firm red tomatoes, diced
^{1}/$_4$ cup finely chopped red onion
1 small garlic clove, finely chopped
1 red or green fresh chile, such as jalapeño, serrano, or
   mirasol, seeded and minced
^{1}/$_3$ cup fresh cilantro leaves, chopped
1 to 2 tablespoons fresh lime juice
^{1}/$_4$ teaspoon salt
^{1}/$_4$ teaspoon ground black pepper

In a medium bowl, combine the tomatillos, tomatoes, onion, garlic, and chile. Let stand at room temperature for 1 hour.

Stir in the cilantro, lime juice, and salt and pepper.

(This salsa can be stored in a tightly sealed container in the refrigerator for up to 4 days.)

Calories: 9.9 kcal
Fat: 0.2 g
Protein: 0.3 g
Carbohydrates: 2.0 g
Sodium: 30.9 mg

black bean dip

MAKES 1^1/2 CUPS; 12 (2-TABLESPOON) SERVINGS

1 (15-ounce) can no-sodium black beans, rinsed and drained
^{1}/2 cup fresh cilantro leaves
^{1}/4 cup chopped red onion
1 garlic clove, finely chopped
2 tablespoons fresh lime juice
1 tablespoon orange juice
1 tablespoon extra-virgin olive oil
^{1}/2 teaspoon minced, canned chipotle chile in adobo
^{1}/4 teaspoon salt

In the work bowl of a food processor, place the beans, cilantro leaves, onion, garlic, lime juice, orange juice, olive oil, chile, and salt. Process until the dip is smooth and creamy, scraping down the sides of the bowl once or twice or as needed.

(The dip can be stored in a tightly sealed container in the refrigerator for up to 4 days.)

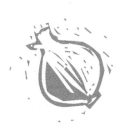

Calories: 40.9 kcal
Fat: 1.2 g
Protein: 2.0 g
Carbohydrates: 5.71 g
Sodium: 45.1 mg

trail mix MAKES ³/4 CUP; 4 SERVINGS

Calories: 178.0 kcal
Fat: 12.5 g
Protein: 5.0 g
Carbohydrates: 13.3 g
Sodium: 1.6 mg

¹/4 cup (1 ounce) raw almonds
¹/4 cup (1 ounce) raw pepitas or sunflower seeds
¹/4 cup (1 ounce) 70% cocoa mini chocolate chips

In a small bowl, combine the almonds, pepitas, and chocolate chips. (Trail mix can be stored in an airtight container for up to 1 week.)

HEALTH BENEFITS:
Anti-Cancer Heart Healthy Boosts Immunity Boosts Metabolism Improves Digestion Miscellaneous

spiced roasted almonds

MAKES 2 CUPS; 16 SERVINGS

2 cups natural whole almonds
1 teaspoon extra-virgin olive oil
3/4 teaspoon ground cumin
3/4 teaspoon ground coriander
¹/4 teaspoon cayenne pepper
Pinch of smoked paprika
¹/2 teaspoon salt
1/8 teaspoon ground black pepper

Preheat the oven to 300°F.

Calories: 105.8 kcal
Fat: 9.3 g
Protein: 3.8 g
Carbohydrates: 3.6 g
Sodium: 60.4 mg

Place the almonds in a large mixing bowl. Add the olive oil, cumin, coriander, cayenne pepper, smoked paprika, and salt and black pepper. Stir until the nuts are thoroughly coated with the oil and spices. Transfer the nuts to a rimmed baking sheet and spread in a single layer.

Bake until lightly toasted, about 25 minutes. Transfer to a large platter to cool completely. (Store almonds in an airtight container for up to 3 days.)

desserts

PEAR SORBET

CHOCOLATE-CINNAMON FROZEN BANANA POPS

ORANGES WITH LEMON-VANILLA YOGURT CREAM

POMEGRANATE-PEAR SALAD

GOLDEN APPLE CRISP

MAPLE-GLAZED PLANTAINS

SPICED FIG AND APPLE COMPOTE

HONEY-GINGER PLUMS

RICE PUDDING

WALNUT-ORANGE CAKE WITH SWEET YOGURT

FUDGE BROWNIES

ALMOND-CHOCOLATE BLONDIES

pear sorbet   MAKES ABOUT 5 CUPS; SERVES 10

$1/2$ cup plus 2 tablespoons honey
4 large organic pears (about 2 pounds), peeled, cored,
    and coarsely chopped (about 4 cups)
1 tablespoon fresh lemon juice
$3/4$ cup ruby port wine
2 tablespoons balsamic vinegar
1 (3-inch) cinnamon stick
1 star anise
Thinly sliced pear, for serving (optional)

In a small saucepan, place $1/2$ cup of the honey and $1/2$ cup water and heat over medium heat. Bring to a boil. Reduce the heat and simmer for 1 minute. Remove from the heat and let cool completely.

In the work bowl of a food processor, pulse the pears and lemon juice until finely chopped. Add the cooled honey mixture and process until smooth. Chill until very cold, at least 4 hours.

Meanwhile, make the sauce (see Note). In a small saucepan, place the port, vinegar, remaining 2 tablespoons honey, the cinnamon stick, and the star anise. Bring to a boil. Reduce the heat to low and simmer until the syrup has thickened and reduced to about $1/3$ cup, about 30 minutes. (Watch the pan carefully during the last 5 to 10 minutes of cooking; it can very quickly go from perfect to burned and bitter.) Remove from the heat and let cool to room temperature before serving; remove and discard the cinnamon stick and star anise.

When the pear puree is cold, freeze it in an ice cream maker according to the manufacturer's directions. The sorbet is best served at once, but it may be transferred to a freezer-safe container and frozen until ready to serve. Let stand at room temperature for 15 minutes before serving.

If not using an ice cream maker, transfer the cold pear puree to a shallow glass or stainless-steel dish. Cover and place in the freezer until frozen solid, about 6 hours. Let the frozen mixture stand at room temperature for 10 minutes. With a large metal spoon, break the puree up into smaller pieces. Transfer the mixture to the work bowl of a food processor. Process until smooth and creamy, occasionally scraping down the sides of the bowl. Serve immediately or place back into the freezer for up to 1 hour before serving. The sorbet will freeze solid but it can simply be processed again until creamy just before serving.

To serve, scoop the sorbet into individual serving bowls and drizzle the syrup over each. Garnish with pear slices if desired.

Note: The sauce can be made ahead of time. Just transfer it to a glass measuring cup and let stand at room temperature for several hours, or for longer storage, cover and refrigerate. Before serving, heat in a microwave oven on high power for a few seconds, just until liquid and pourable.

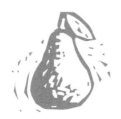

Calories: 143.0 kcal
Fat: 0.1 g
Protein: 0.5 g
Carbohydrates: 32.9 g
Sodium: 4.0 mg

MASTERING FRUITS
Smart Selection

As with vegetables, do not buy fruits precut, and be sure to pick fruits with rich color. Respected physician and culinary wizard Dr. John La Puma, otherwise known as ChefMD, likes to say that strong color means strong medicine.

Ripe fruit is best. When fruits are eaten green, their vitamins and phytonutrients haven't had the appropriate time to mature. Some fruits must be picked ripe and others can ripen after being picked. Here are some rules to guide you:

- Tropical fruits like banana, papaya, and mango can ripen at home if they have not been picked too early. Wait to consume them until they are slightly soft to the touch and have a full, rich aroma.
- Pineapples and melons should be picked and consumed ripe. They don't ripen after being picked. For melons, look for a smooth rind that isn't overly dull or shiny. Smell the fruit. It should be fragrant and smell like itself, not the cardboard it was shipped in. Avoid melons that do not have a round spot on the bottom. That usually means they have been harvested prematurely.
- Grapes and berries should be picked and consumed ripe, but not soggy or mushy, dry, or wrinkled. Make sure the color of the berries is deep and dark, which indicates they are ripe. Studies have shown that the smaller the berries, the more nutrients and flavor they contain.
- Thin-skinned fruits like apples, pears, peaches, plums, and kiwi should be picked as close to ripe as possible. Avoid soft spots, punctures, or bruises on the fruit. These are usually signs of decay.
- Thick-skinned citrus fruits can be picked before they've ripened or when ripe. Look for a thinner-skinned fruit, as it means more juice and pulp. Avoid fruits that are overly ripe or have hard patches or "scalds." They can give the fruit a moldy taste.

Smart Storage

Different fruits have different storage requirements. Here are some easy guidelines to follow:

- Buy melons and tropical fruits within a day or two of when you plan to eat them. They should be kept at room temperature because they can lose their flavor when stored in the fridge. You can refrigerate them for 20 minutes before you eat them, if you prefer the taste of the fruit cold, but not before then.

- Grapes and berries should be refrigerated as soon as you bring them home; grapes can last up to 2 days, berries up to 1 day in the refrigerator.
- Thin-skinned fruits like apples, peaches, pears, kiwi, plums, and nectarines can be put in the fridge or stored in a paper bag at room temperature. The key here is whether or not you like your fruit cold and how quickly you want it to ripen. Apples can be stored in the refrigerator for several weeks or at room temperature for up to 4 days. Other thin-skinned fruit can be stored in the refrigerator for 3 to 4 days or at room temperature for 2 to 3 days.
- Citrus fruits like oranges, grapefruits, lemons, and limes can be stored at room temperature or refrigerated, depending on how long it will be before you consume the fruit. Room-temperature citrus will last for up to 5 days, while refrigerated citrus will last for up to 10 days. Citrus stored at room temperature will be juicier. Be sure to give your citrus fruits space. If stored on top of each other, they will rot sooner, as they give off a gas when they ripen, and the collective gas from multiple fruits speeds the process.

Smart Preparation
- Always wash fruit, even if you aren't eating the skin or rind. When you cut into it you want to be sure no dirt or toxins get inside. Rinse under cold water just before you eat, not before, as excess water can stay on fruit and make it moldy.
- Remove tops, caps, or stems *after* washing so excess water doesn't seep into the fruit along with pesticides or fungus that might be lingering on its outside.
- Cut your fruit only right before you plan on eating it. Air oxidizes fruit and compromises its nutrients.
- If you must store cut fruit, put it in an airtight container and refrigerate. You can also store fruit for several hours by submerging it in cold water; add a tablespoon of lemon, orange, or lime juice for every cup of water. The vitamin C in the juice acts as an antioxidant and helps prevent browning.
- Unlike vegetables, fruits are best eaten raw or very lightly cooked. Most of the vitamins, antioxidants, and enzymes in fruit are unable to withstand high cooking temperatures.

chocolate-cinnamon frozen banana pops

This is an entirely grown-up version of kiddie banana-chocolate pops. And they not only taste great but also have all the heart-healthy benefits that come from key ingredients. How's that for being young at heart?

To have sufficient chocolate to properly dip the bananas, you need to melt enough to form a good puddle. Spread whatever melted chocolate you have left over on waxed paper and let it stand until hardened. Then break or chop it up and store in an airtight container. Sprinkle a little on nonfat Greek yogurt for a nice chocolate kick. SERVES 6

2 bananas, peeled and cut crosswise into thirds
8 ounces 70% cocoa chocolate, chopped
1/2 teaspoon ground cinnamon
1/4 cup chopped hazelnuts, toasted (page 96)

Line a baking sheet with wax paper. Insert a popsicle stick or wooden skewer in one end of each banana piece. Freeze until hard, at least 2 hours.

When ready to dip the bananas, place the chocolate and cinnamon in a heatproof bowl set over—not in—a pan of gently simmering water. Stir just until melted. Make sure no water gets into the chocolate or it will "seize up," becoming clumpy, oily, and unusable.

Have ready a baking sheet lined with wax paper. Work with one banana piece at a time and leave the remaining bananas in the freezer. Dip the banana in the chocolate, spooning on additional chocolate to cover. Sprinkle the banana with hazelnuts and set it on the prepared baking sheet. Repeat with the remaining bananas. Place the baking sheet in the freezer until ready to serve or for up to 2 days (cover if storing longer than a few hours). Let stand at room temperature for 5 minutes before serving.

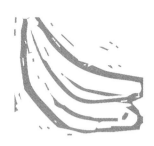

Calories: 153.7 kcal
Fat: 8.4 g
Protein: 2.4 g
Carbohydrates: 20.7g
Sodium: 0.5 mg

HEALTH BENEFITS:
Boosts Immunity Boosts Metabolism Strong Bones Improves Digestion Healthy Skin

oranges with lemon-vanilla yogurt cream SERVES 2

3 tablespoons low-fat vanilla or plain Greek yogurt
1^1/2 teaspoons fresh lemon juice
2 tablespoons honey, if using plain yogurt
^{1}/4 teaspoon pure vanilla extract, if using plain yogurt
2 medium oranges, peeled and separated into segments
^{1}/2 teaspoon grated lemon zest

Calories: 149.3 kcal
Fat: 0.6 g
Protein: 3.2 g
Carbohydrates: 35.9 g
Sodium: 9.2 mg

In a small mixing bowl, blend the yogurt and lemon juice. If using plain yogurt, add the honey and vanilla.

Divide the orange segments between two small serving bowls. Pour over the yogurt cream and garnish with the grated lemon zest. Serve.

HEALTH BENEFITS:
Anti-Cancer Heart Healthy Boosts Metabolism Anti-Inflammatory Healthy Skin

pomegranate-pear salad SERVES 2

1 tangerine, peeled and separated into segments
^{1}/2 ripe pear, cored and chopped
^{1}/2 cup pomegranate seeds (see page 135)
^{1}/4 cup walnuts, toasted (page 96)
2 tablespoons honey

Calories: 231.3 kcal
Fat: 10.1 g
Protein: 3.3 g
Carbohydrates: 36.9 g
Sodium: 3.1 mg

In a small mixing bowl, combine the tangerine segments, pear, pomegranate seeds, and walnuts. Toss gently to combine. Divide between two serving bowls. Drizzle 1 tablespoon honey over each bowl. Serve.

golden apple crisp SERVES 8

$^1/_4$ cup virgin coconut oil

$^1/_4$ cup honey

4 Golden Delicious apples (about 2 pounds), peeled, cored, and cut
   into $^3/_4$-inch chunks (about 6 cups)

1 tablespoon fresh lemon juice

1 tablespoon plus $^1/_2$ cup white whole-wheat flour

1 cup rolled oats (not instant)

1 tablespoon finely chopped walnuts

$^1/_2$ teaspoon ground cinnamon

$^1/_4$ teaspoon grated nutmeg

$^1/_4$ teaspoon salt

8 tablespoons low-fat plain Greek yogurt

Preheat the oven to 375°F.

Into a glass measuring cup, put the oil and honey. Microwave on high power until melted, about 30 seconds, stirring once or twice.

In a large mixing bowl, place the apples and add the lemon juice and 1 tablespoon flour. Toss to coat. Transfer the fruit to a 1$^1/_2$-quart baking dish and spread evenly.

In a medium bowl, combine the remaining $^1/_2$ cup flour, the rolled oats, walnuts, cinnamon, nutmeg, and salt. Stir with a fork until the ingredients are well combined. Pour in the oil and honey, and stir until the mixture is well blended and crumbly. Use your fingers to distribute the crumbs evenly over the fruit.

Bake until the topping is golden brown and the apples are bubbling, about 50 minutes. Let the crisp cool for about 15 minutes before serving.

Spoon the warm crisp into eight serving dishes. Top each serving with a spoonful of yogurt and serve.

Calories: 213.1 kcal

Fat: 8.6 g

Protein: 4.4 g

Carbohydrates: 32.5 g

Sodium: 67.3 mg

maple-glazed plantains

Support men's reproductive health: It turns out that maple syrup reduces prostate size and boosts reproductive hormones.

Plantains can be used at every stage of ripeness, from green and underripe, when they are used for savory dishes, to yellow and almost black, when they are sweeter and good for dessert. For this dish, use a plantain that is at least ripe enough to be completely yellow with some black spots, or even one that is very ripe and completely black. SERVES 4

1 ripe plantain
1 cup low-fat plain Greek yogurt
2 teaspoons virgin coconut oil
1^1/2 tablespoons maple syrup

Place the plantain on a cutting board and use a sharp knife to slice off both ends. Use the knife to make a cut all the way down the inside curve of the plantain; cut the skin just deeply enough to reach the flesh, but not so deep that you slice the flesh. Gently pull off and discard the peel. Cut the plantain into 1/4-inch-thick rounds.

Divide the yogurt among four small serving bowls. Set aside in the fridge to keep it cold.

In a large, cast-iron skillet, heat the oil over medium-high heat. Add the plantain slices and cook until browned, about 1 minute. Turn and cook for 30 seconds, until beginning to brown on the underside. Drizzle the maple syrup over the plantains and cook until caramelized and syrupy, about 1 minute. Remove from the heat and immediately divide the plantains among the four dishes, spooning some syrup over each serving. Enjoy.

Calories: 118.2 kcal
Fat: 3.6 g
Protein: 5.3 g
Carbohydrates: 18.2 g
Sodium: 20.8 mg

spiced fig and apple compote Serve

this warm or at room temperature, on its own or over

Greek yogurt. SERVES 4

2 quarter-size thin slices fresh ginger
5 whole cloves
1 (4-inch) cinnamon stick
2 medium Golden Delicious apples, peeled, cored, and
    cut into $^1/_2$-inch cubes
$^1/_2$ cup fresh orange juice
2 tablespoons honey
8 ounces fresh figs, trimmed and quartered
$^1/_4$ cup walnuts, toasted (page 96)

Lay a double layer of cheesecloth on your work surface and place in its center the ginger, cloves, and cinnamon. Enclose the spices and tie with kitchen string to form a spice bundle. (Alternatively, just throw it all loose into the saucepan, but don't forget to use a slotted spoon to fish out the spices after cooking unless you *want* to bite into a whole clove.)

In a small saucepan, place the apples, orange juice, honey, and spice bundle. Bring to a boil. Reduce the heat and simmer until the liquid has reduced by half, about 10 minutes.

Stir in the figs and simmer gently for 5 minutes.

Remove the pan from the heat. Remove and discard the spice bundle. Stir in the nuts. Serve warm or at room temperature. (You can store the compote in a tightly sealed container in the refrigerator for up to 4 days. Heat in a microwave for about 30 seconds on high power, stirring once during heating, or in a small saucepan before serving. Add a teaspoon or two of water to the saucepan if the compote seems dry.)

Calories: 169.1 kcal
Fat: 5.0 g
Protein: 2.0 g
Carbohydrates: 31.6 g
Sodium: 2.1 mg

HEALTH BENEFITS:

Heart Healthy Boosts Immunity Boosts Metabolism Strong Bones Anti-Inflammatory Miscellaneous

honey-ginger plums
Briefly roasting plums with honey, ginger, and cinnamon makes your kitchen smell heavenly and transforms the fruit into an addictive dessert elegant enough to serve guests. When summer ends and fall comes, prepare pears in the same way. SERVES 4

2 tablespoons chopped Brazil nuts
$1/3$ cup honey
3 quarter-size thin slices fresh ginger
1 (3-inch) cinnamon stick
4 ripe plums, pitted and quartered, or 2 ripe, firm pears, cored and cut into 8 wedges
$1/2$ cup low-fat plain Greek yogurt

Preheat the oven to 350°F.

Spread the nuts on a rimmed baking sheet. Toast in the oven until lightly browned and fragrant, 4 to 5 minutes. Immediately transfer to a plate to cool.

Meanwhile, in a cast-iron skillet big enough to hold the fruit wedges in a single layer, stir together the honey, ginger slices, cinnamon stick, and $1/3$ cup water. Heat over medium heat until the liquid comes to a simmer. Add the plum or pear wedges. Place in the oven and bake for 15 minutes. Use a fork or thin spatula to flip the fruit over and bake until the fruit is softened and the liquid is syrupy, about 15 minutes.

Divide the yogurt among four small bowls. Spoon over the plums or pears with their syrup. Sprinkle each serving with nuts and serve.

CHOOSING HONEY
Honey is loaded with vitamins, minerals, amino acids, and antioxidants, and is a great source of vitamin B_6, but not when it's been filtered, like the kind you find at your local supermarket. Go with darker colored honey for its additional antioxidants, and whenever possible, choose raw honey for its optimal health benefits.

Calories: 162.9 kcal
Fat: 3.7 g
Protein: 3.7 g
Carbohydrates: 31.9 g
Sodium: 10.3 mg

rice pudding SERVES 4

3^1/2 cups almond milk
^{1}/2 cup coconut milk
^{1}/2 cup short-grain brown rice
2 tablespoons agave syrup
1 lime
1 large orange

In a medium saucepan, stir together the almond milk, coconut milk, rice, and agave syrup. Bring to a boil over medium-high heat. Reduce the heat to low, cover, and simmer very gently, stirring occasionally, until the rice is tender but chewy and has absorbed most of the liquid, about 1^1/2 hours.

Meanwhile, finely grate the zest from the lime and the orange. Transfer each to a small bowl, cover, and place in the refrigerator until needed.

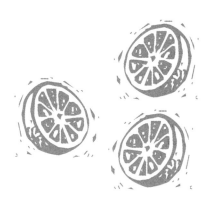

Squeeze 1 tablespoon of juice from the lime and set the juice aside. Use a sharp, thin-bladed knife to cut just enough of the top and bottom off the orange to expose its flesh. Set the orange cut side down on a cutting board and slice off the peel and pith, following the curve of the fruit with the knife. Holding the peeled fruit over a bowl to catch any juice, cut the segments away from the thin membranes holding them together and set them aside on a plate. When all the segments have been cut away, hold the remaining pith and membrane over the bowl and squeeze any remaining juice from it. Set aside the fruit and juice separately.

When the rice pudding is cooked, remove the pan from the heat and stir in the lime juice and the orange juice. Let stand for about 10 minutes.

Divide the orange pieces among four small serving dishes. Spoon the rice pudding over. Sprinkle each serving with a pinch each of the orange zest and the lime zest. Serve.

Calories: 252.8 kcal

Fat: 9.2 g

Protein: 3.8 g

Carbohydrates: 40.6 g

Sodium: 138.0 mg

walnut-orange cake with sweet yogurt This

wonderfully moist and not overly sweet cake is bursting with the flavor of
toasted walnuts and orange. Grate the zest from the oranges before you juice
them for the cake. SERVES 14 TO 16

1^1/2 cups chopped walnuts, toasted (page 96)
1 cup white whole-wheat flour, plus more for the pan
2 teaspoons aluminum-free baking powder
^{1}/4 teaspoon baking soda
^{1}/2 teaspoon salt
1 tablespoon plus 1 teaspoon grated orange zest, plus
    more for garnish
3/4 cup fresh orange juice
^{1}/2 cup olive oil, plus more for the pan
^{1}/2 cup plus 1 teaspoon mild honey, such as clover or
    orange blossom
2 large eggs, at room temperature
1 cup low-fat plain Greek yogurt

Preheat the oven to 350°F. Brush a 9-inch springform pan with olive
oil and add a couple spoonfuls of flour. Rotate the pan and tap its
sides to thoroughly coat the bottom and sides with flour. Tap out
the excess. Set aside.

In the work bowl of a food processor, place the walnuts. Pulse
them in 1- or 2-second bursts until they are finely ground; do not
overprocess or they will become overly oily. Transfer the nuts to
a large bowl. Add the flour, baking powder, baking soda, salt, and
1 tablespoon orange zest. Whisk until well combined.

In a medium bowl, place the orange juice, olive oil, $1/2$ cup honey, and the eggs. Whisk until well combined. Pour the liquid ingredients over the dry ingredients and stir just until moistened. Do not overmix.

Pour the batter into the prepared pan and bake until the top springs back when gently pressed with your fingertip and the edges are pulling away from the pan, about 40 minutes. Transfer the pan to a cooling rack and let cool for 10 minutes. Run a thin knife around the outside of the cake and remove the sides. Let cool completely.

If you wish to unmold the cake from the bottom of the pan, have a cake serving plate ready. Run a thin spatula or knife under the cake to loosen it from the cake base. Place a cooling rack over the cake and flip it over. Lift the cake base off the cake and place the cake serving plate upside down over the cake. Flip the rack, cake, and plate over and lift off the rack.

While the cake is baking, in a small bowl, place the yogurt, remaining 1 teaspoon honey, and remaining 1 teaspoon grated orange zest. Gently stir together until well combined. Refrigerate until needed.

Serve each slice of cake with a spoonful of yogurt and garnished with a pinch of orange zest.

Calories: 248.5 kcal
Fat: 17.5 g
Protein: 5.5 g
Carbohydrates: 20.8 g
Sodium: 185.5 mg

fudge brownies

These brownies are outrageously moist and intensely chocolatey. Whip up a batch the next time you're jonesing for chocolate and you won't be disappointed. MAKES 16 (2-INCH) BROWNIES

Olive oil spray for the pan
$2/3$ cup mild honey, such as clover or orange blossom
$1/3$ cup natural, unsweetened cocoa powder
$1/2$ cup white whole-wheat flour
$1/4$ teaspoon aluminum-free baking powder
$1/4$ teaspoon baking soda
$1/4$ teaspoon salt
$1/2$ cup unsweetened applesauce
2 tablespoons olive oil
1 large egg, at room temperature
$3/4$ teaspoon pure vanilla extract

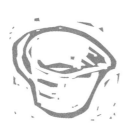

Preheat the oven to 350°F. Spray an 8-inch square pan with olive oil. Set aside.

Place the honey in a large glass measuring cup. Microwave on high power until the honey is runny and just bubbling, 45 to 60 seconds. Add the cocoa and stir with a fork until well combined. Let cool to room temperature.

Meanwhile, in a small bowl, place the flour, baking powder, baking soda, and salt. Whisk until well combined.

In a large bowl, combine the applesauce, oil, egg, and vanilla. Whisk together until well blended. Add the honey-cocoa mixture and whisk until smooth. Add the flour mixture to the liquid mixture and stir until no traces of flour remain. Scrape the batter into the prepared pan.

Bake until the surface looks dry around the edges of the pan and a toothpick inserted in the center comes out with moist crumbs clinging to it, about 25 minutes. Do not overbake. Place the pan on a cooling rack and let cool completely before slicing into 16 squares. (Store the brownies in an airtight container at room temperature for up to 3 days.)

Calories: 86.2 kcal
Fat: 2.2 g
Protein: 1.3 g
Carbohydrates: 16.0 g
Sodium: 63.6 mg

Anti-Cancer Heart Healthy Boosts Metabolism Improves Mood Healthy Skin

almond-chocolate blondies

MAKES 20 (1^1/2 BY 2-INCH) BLONDIES

Olive oil spray for the pan
1 cup almond butter
^{2}/3 cup honey, such as clover or orange blossom
^{1}/4 cup coconut milk
3 large eggs, at room temperature
2 teaspoons pure vanilla extract
^{3}/4 cup white whole-wheat flour
^{3}/4 cup ground flaxseed
^{3}/4 teaspoon aluminum-free baking powder
^{1}/4 teaspoon baking soda
^{3}/4 cup 70% cocoa mini chocolate chunks

Preheat the oven to 350°F. Spray an 8-inch square glass baking dish with olive oil.

In a large bowl, place the almond butter, honey, coconut milk, eggs, and vanilla. Whisk together until well blended and smooth.

In a separate bowl, place the flour, flaxseed, baking powder, and baking soda. Whisk together until well mixed. Add the dry ingredients to the almond butter mixture and stir just until blended. Then stir in the chocolate chunks.

Scrape the batter into the prepared dish and bake until browned around the edges and a toothpick comes out with moist crumbs clinging to it, about 35 minutes. Transfer the baking pan to a cooling rack and let cool for about 15 minutes before cutting. Cut into 20 squares and serve. (The blondies can be stored in an airtight container at room temperature for up to 3 days.)

Calories: 212.1 kcal
Fat: 13.0 g
Protein: 5.0 g
Carbohydrates: 22.0 g
Sodium: 103.3 mg

basics

....

poached chicken

This is just about the simplest way to prepare chicken breast, and once it's cooked you can use it warm or cold in a multitude of ways. In this book alone there's a Chicken Salad with Red Grapes and Toasted Pecans (page 109) recipe and one for Healthy Cobb Salad (page 100), but this is the kind of basic ingredient that you can make once and use all week. Shred it over any salad or vegetarian soup to add a bit of protein. Slice or shred it and roll it up in a whole-wheat tortilla with a couple spoonfuls of Tomatillo and Tomato Salsa (page 234) and a couple of thin slices of avocado. Or serve it as is, topped with a spoonful of Fruit Vinaigrette (page 263) or Simple Marinara Sauce (page 266) alongside a basic cooked vegetable. SERVES 4

1 pound boneless, skinless chicken breast
2 to 3 strips lemon zest, removed with a vegetable peeler
1 fresh or dried bay leaf

Place the chicken in a shallow pan with a tight-fitting lid. Fill the pan with water to cover the chicken by about 1^{1}/2 inches. Add the lemon zest and bay leaf, and set the pan over medium heat. Bring the water to a simmer, then reduce the heat so the water barely bubbles, partially cover, and cook until the meat is firm and releases clear juices when pierced with a fork, about 10 minutes.

Remove the chicken from the water and transfer it to a towel-lined plate to drain. Serve warm or let cool completely. Store in a tightly sealed container in the refrigerator for up to 4 days.

Calories: 121.6 kcal
Fat: 2.6 g
Protein: 22.9 g
Carbohydrates: 0 g
Sodium: 54.5 mg

hard-boiled eggs

Eggs are a nearly perfect food, containing almost every essential vitamin and mineral our bodies need. Eating an egg every day is not a bad idea, and this super-easy method of cooking them makes it a breeze to whip up a half dozen or so and keep them in the fridge all week long, so there will always be one available at snack time or for the Healthy Cobb Salad (page 100), or Mediterranean Tuna Salad Rolls (page 107). It's a little strange that they're called hard-*boiled* eggs, however. You should *never* boil an egg—unless you like them rubbery. Check out this foolproof method for perfect eggs every time. Let the eggs stand at room temperature for about 45 minutes before cooking. If your eggs are just out of the fridge, add 3 minutes to the "cooking" time, for a total of 13 minutes.

6 large eggs, at cool room temperature

In a large saucepan, place the eggs in a single layer. Add water to cover by 1 inch. Cover and heat over medium-high heat just until the water comes to a boil. Immediately remove the pan from the heat; leave the cover in place. Let stand for 10 minutes.

Meanwhile, prepare a bowl of ice water. When the eggs are cooked, immediately transfer them to the ice water and let stand until completely cool.

For easy shelling, tap the eggs on the counter and start shelling at the wide end. Doing so under a gentle stream of cold, running water easily removes any small bits of shell.

Store unshelled cooked eggs in the refrigerator for up to 1 week (mark them with a pencil—so you know which are cooked—and put them back in their carton for easiest storage).

Calories: 70.0 kcal
Fat: 4.5 g
Protein: 6.0 g
Carbohydrates: 1.0 g
Sodium: 65.0 mg

black beans Cooking your own black beans is far cheaper, tastier, and healthier than using any canned type. Cooked beans can be stored for several days in the refrigerator or for months in the freezer, so it's never a bad idea to whip up a batch for storage. The main issue with cooking beans is that you can never be entirely certain how long they'll take to cook because the age of the bean is a major factor there: the older the bean, the longer it takes to cook. It's best to buy your beans someplace where you know there's rapid turnover; otherwise, that bag you buy may have been sitting there for months. MAKES ABOUT 6 CUPS

> 1 pound dried black beans (about 2^1/2 cups)
> ^{1}/2 teaspoon salt

Place the beans in a strainer and pick through them, discarding any debris. Rinse well. Transfer the beans to a large saucepan and add cold water to cover by about 1 inch. Bring to a boil over high heat. Reduce the heat, partially cover, and cook until tender to the bite but still holding their shape, 1 to 2 hours, stirring occasionally. Stir in the salt.

Drain and cool if using immediately. Otherwise, transfer the beans and their cooking liquid to a tightly sealed container and store in the refrigerator for up to 3 days or in the freezer for up to 6 months.

Calories: 128.9 kcal
Fat: 0.5 g
Protein: 8.2 g
Carbohydrates: 23.6 g
Sodium: 41.9 mg

HEALTH BENEFITS:
Anti-Cancer Heart Healthy Boosts Metabolism Miscellaneous

brown rice MAKES ABOUT 3 CUPS; SERVES 4

$1/8$ teaspoon salt
1 cup long-grain or short-grain brown rice

In a medium saucepan, bring 2 cups water and the salt to a boil. Stir in the rice. Reduce the heat, cover, and simmer gently until tender, 45 to 50 minutes. Let stand, covered, for 10 minutes. Remove the cover and fluff with a fork. Serve.

Calories: 171.1 kcal
Fat: 1.4 g
Protein: 3.7 g
Carbohydrates: 35.7 g
Sodium: 123.2 mg

HEALTH BENEFITS:
Heart Healthy Boosts Metabolism

couscous MAKES ABOUT 3 CUPS; SERVES 4

$1/8$ teaspoon salt
1 cup whole-wheat couscous

In a small saucepan, bring $1^1/2$ cups water and the salt to a boil. Stir in the couscous, cover, and simmer for 2 minutes. Stir to fluff the couscous, then cover and remove from the heat. Let stand, covered, for 5 minutes. Fluff with a fork and serve.

Calories: 105.0 kcal
Fat: 0.5 g
Protein: 4.0 g
Carbohydrates: 22.5 g
Sodium: 120.0 mg

HEALTH BENEFITS:
Heart Healthy Boosts Metabolism Miscellaneous

quinoa   MAKES ABOUT 3¹/2 CUPS; SERVES 4

^{1}/8 teaspoon salt
1 cup quinoa

In a small saucepan, bring 2 cups water and the salt to a boil.

Meanwhile, place the quinoa in a strainer and rinse under cold running water until the rinse water runs clear. Stir the quinoa into the boiling water, cover, and simmer until the quinoa is tender and the water is absorbed, about 15 minutes. Let stand, covered, for 5 minutes. Fluff with a fork and serve.

Calories: 159.0 kcal
Fat: 2.5 g
Protein: 5.6 g
Carbohydrates: 29.3 g
Sodium: 128.9 mg

fruit vinaigrette
This sweet-and-savory vinaigrette is my favorite because it's so versatile—just use whatever soft fruit you have. It's a great dressing for a salad of greens (add more water to make a thinner vinaigrette for delicate greens such as baby leaves) or chopped vegetables, or spoon a little on top of grilled fish or poultry. Add a spoonful of chopped scallion greens or snipped chives for a bit of a kick. MAKES ABOUT 3/4 CUP; 6 (2-TABLESPOON) SERVINGS

1 cup chopped fruit, such as pineapple, mango, blueberries,
    raspberries, orange, tangerine, or grapefruit
1 tablespoon extra-virgin olive oil
1 teaspoon balsamic vinegar

In a blender, place the fruit, olive oil, vinegar, and up to 2 teaspoons water. Blend until smooth and pourable, adding more water 1 teaspoon at a time as necessary to thin the mixture. Use at once or store in a tightly covered container in the refrigerator for up to 3 days.

Calories: 34.0 kcal
Fat: 2.4 g
Protein: 0.1 g
Carbohydrates: 3.4 g
Sodium: 0.5 mg

vegetable broth   I know that asking you to make your own broth may seem a little over the top, but believe me, in the case of vegetable broth, it's worth it. While you can find some decent low-sodium chicken broth on the market, store-bought vegetable broth is mostly awful and often full of sodium. Homemade vegetable broth doesn't take long to make—don't let the veggies simmer longer than an hour, for best flavor—and keeps for months in the freezer. The broth adds flavor and depth to any soup. Divide it into 2-cup containers, if you like, and use it in place of water to cook any grain, including the Barley Risotto with Asparagus and Lemon (page 196).

You can treat this recipe as more of a suggestion than a hard-and-fast rule. A great way to make vegetable broth is to simply save a bag of vegetable trimmings in your freezer. Whenever you prepare any vegetable for cooking, toss the extras in there. Cook the recipes in this book, and in no time you'll have a bag full of asparagus ends, leek or scallion greens, mushroom stems, fennel fronds, carrot peels, celery ends, parsley stems, even ginger trimmings if you want to add an Asian note—all the makings for a perfectly delicious vegetable broth. Pop them in a pot with an onion, garlic if you like it, and a carrot for sweetness. Cover with cold water and continue as directed below. Talk about cheap and easy!

Stay away from eggplant and cruciferous vegetables such as cabbage, broccoli, cauliflower, brussels sprouts, kale, and collard greens, however, because they can overwhelm the flavor of stock.

There is no nutritional analysis of this recipe because it really does depend on what you put in the pot. Rest assured that as long as you follow these guidelines, the result will be a very low-sodium, nutritionally beneficial addition wherever you use it.

MAKES ABOUT 2 QUARTS

> 1 large yellow or red onion, peeled if desired (the peel will add color) and quartered
> 1 garlic clove, peeled and halved (optional)
> 2 large carrots, cut into 2-inch pieces
> 2 celery stalks, cut into 2-inch pieces
> 8 ounces button or cremini mushrooms, coarsely chopped
> 2 small turnips or 1 fennel bulb, coarsely chopped
> 6 fresh parsley sprigs
> 4 fresh thyme sprigs
> 1 fresh or dried bay leaf

In a stockpot, place the onion, garlic, carrots, celery, mushrooms, and turnips. Tie the parsley, thyme, and bay leaf together with kitchen string and add to the pot. Add 2 quarts cold water, or enough to cover the vegetables. Partially cover the pot and bring the water to a boil over medium-high heat. Reduce the heat and skim any foam from the surface. Simmer gently, partially covered, for 1 hour.

Strain the broth through a fine-mesh strainer; do not press on the vegetables or the broth will be very cloudy. Let cool to room temperature. Store in a tightly sealed container for up to 3 days in the refrigerator or in the freezer for up to 6 months.

simple marinara sauce

Store-bought marinara sauce might seem like a safe cheat, but so many are loaded with sugar and even high-fructose corn syrup that it's really anything but. Making marinara sauce at home is not only cheaper but also allows you to control everything that goes into it—plus it's easy! Marinara stores beautifully (see below) and actually gets better with age as the flavors meld and mellow. So make a batch when you have a spare half hour on the weekend and serve some of it with the Quinoa-Stuffed Peppers (page 200). Then refrigerate the rest to serve a few days later over whole-wheat linguine or a poached chicken breast. Or make a lunch of a small portion of leftover Barley Risotto with Asparagus and Lemon (page 196) with a little marinara spooned over it.

MAKES ABOUT 4 CUPS; SERVES 8

1 tablespoon olive oil
1 cup finely chopped red onion
2 garlic cloves, finely chopped
1 fresh or dried bay leaf
$^1/_4$ cup tomato paste
1 (28-ounce) can low-sodium crushed tomatoes
1 tablespoon chopped fresh parsley, or 1 teaspoon dried
1 tablespoon chopped fresh oregano, or 1 teaspoon dried
1 tablespoon chopped fresh basil, or 1 teaspoon dried
1 teaspoon balsamic vinegar
$^1/_4$ teaspoon salt
$^1/_4$ teaspoon ground black pepper

In a large skillet or other heavy-bottomed pan, heat the olive oil over medium-low heat. Add the onion, garlic, and bay leaf, and cook, stirring, until softened and just beginning to brown, 6 to 8 minutes.

Push the onion and garlic to one side of the pan and add the tomato paste to the cleared spot. Cook for about 2 minutes. Stir the onion and garlic into the paste and continue to cook, stirring occasionally, until the paste is darker in color, 2 to 3 minutes.

Stir in the crushed tomatoes, parsley, oregano, basil, vinegar, and salt and pepper. Increase the heat to medium and bring to a boil. Reduce the heat and simmer for 15 minutes. Remove and discard the bay leaf.

If a very smooth sauce is desired, transfer the sauce to the work bowl of a food processor or a blender and process until smooth. Otherwise, leave it be.

Serve warm. For longer storage, let the sauce cool and transfer it to a tightly sealed container. Store in the refrigerator for up to 4 days or freeze for up to 6 months.

Calories: 53.2 kcal
Fat: 1.8 g
Protein: 1.4 g
Carbohydrates: 7.2 g
Sodium: 161.9 mg

HEALTH BENEFITS:
Anti-Cancer Heart Healthy Boosts Metabolism

ketchup The taste and texture of most store-bought ketchup brings to mind nothing more than red-colored corn syrup. This ketchup, on the other hand, gets its sweetness from maple syrup; its aroma and flavor from cloves, allspice, and cinnamon; and its texture from fresh, ripe tomatoes. In short, it's nothing at all like that crappy bottled stuff.

MAKES ABOUT 2 CUPS; 32 (1-TABLESPOON) SERVINGS

>   3 tablespoons olive oil, plus more for the pan
>   2 pounds ripe plum tomatoes, cut lengthwise in half
>   1 teaspoon whole allspice
>   1 teaspoon whole cloves
>   1 (3-inch) cinnamon stick
>   1 cup chopped red onion
>   2 garlic cloves, chopped
>   1 tablespoon tomato paste
>   2 tablespoons maple syrup
>   1 tablespoon cider vinegar
>   1/4 teaspoon salt

Set a rack 6 inches below the broiler and heat the broiler to high. Brush a rimmed baking sheet with olive oil.

Place the tomatoes cut side down on the baking sheet. Brush the tomatoes with 2 tablespoons of the olive oil. Broil until they are softened and brown in spots, 8 to 10 minutes. Remove from the oven and set the pan aside.

Meanwhile, lay a double layer of unbleached cheesecloth on the work surface. Place the allspice, cloves, and cinnamon stick in the center. Bundle them in the cheesecloth and tie it tightly with kitchen string. Set aside. Alternatively, you can toss all the spices directly into the pot, but be sure to fish them all out before you puree the ketchup.

In a Dutch oven or other large heavy-bottomed saucepan, heat the remaining 1 tablespoon olive oil over medium-low heat. Add the onion and garlic and cook, stirring occasionally, until softened, about 8 minutes. Stir in the tomato paste and cook, continuing to stir occasionally, for 2 minutes. Add the reserved tomatoes and their juice, the maple syrup, vinegar, salt, and spice bundle. Cover and cook for 5 minutes. Remove the cover and simmer for 30 minutes.

Remove and discard the spice bundle. Transfer the mixture to the work bowl of a food processor or a blender and puree until smooth. Clean out the Dutch oven and return the puree to it. Simmer until thickened and reduced, 50 minutes to 1 hour, stirring occasionally.

Let cool before serving. Store the ketchup in a tightly sealed container in the refrigerator for 1 week or freeze for up to 6 months. For individual portions, freeze in ice cube trays until frozen solid, then transfer to a freezer-safe container and just pop one out whenever you need a little ketchup; let it stand at room temperature for 30 minutes or defrost in the microwave.

Calories: 23.2 kcal
Fat: 1.4 g
Protein: 0.3 g
Carbohydrates: 2.7 g
Sodium: 20.8 mg

RESOURCES

ORGANIZATIONS

Environmental Defense Fund
www.edf.org
A nonprofit organization focused on finding solutions to global warming; protecting our oceans, land, and freshwater ecosystems; and reducing pollution and toxic chemicals. Check them out to learn more about contaminants in fish.

Environmental Protection Agency safe water hotline
800-426-4791
www.epa.gov/safewater
The EPA is charged with the task of keeping the nation's groundwater and drinking water safe. Many local reports are posted regarding drinking water quality; or check them out to find out how to get the report on your local drinking water.

Mothers for Natural Law
www.safe-food.org
Go to their Web site for more information on genetically modified foods.

Monterey Bay Aquarium and Seafood Watch
www.seafoodwatch.org
The Seafood Watch program, run by the Monterey Bay Aquarium, recommends which fish and shellfish to buy and which to avoid, based on whether they are raised or fished under sustainable conditions.

Organic Consumers Association
www.organicconsumers.org
A nonprofit public-interest organization dedicated to issues such as food safety and industrial agriculture. Check out their GreenPeople directory of organic food suppliers.

World's Healthiest Foods
www.whfoods.org
Visit this site for information on healthy food choices.

Environmental Working Group
www.ewg.org
A nonprofit and advocacy group dedicated to educating consumers about issues relating to public health and the environment. Check them out to learn more about pesticides, BPA, drinking water quality, and other environmental concerns.

Organic Grocery Deals
www.organicgrocerydeals.com
A great resource for "clipping" coupons for organic food.

Organic Kitchen
www.organickitchen.com
Visit this site for a list of cyber-markets offering organic products in your area.

Alternative Farming Systems Information Center
afsic.nal.usda.gov
AFSIC is run by the U.S. Department of Agriculture and focuses on topics related to sustainable and alternative farming. Check them out to see what the government is doing to support local, sustainable foods and to find a farmers' market or CSA near you.

Food Routes Network
www.foodroutes.org
FoodRoutes is a nonprofit dedicated to helping organizations that are working to rebuild local, community-based food systems. Use their Eat Well Guide to find local, sustainably produced food.

Local Harvest
www.localharvest.org
This is a nationwide directory of small farms, farmers' markets, and other local food sources; use them to find a farmers' market or CSA near you.

Cooperative Grocer
www.cooperativegrocer.coop/coops
A great place to visit to find a food co-op near you.

Cooperative Grocers' Information Network
www.cgin.coop
To get information on starting a co-op in your area, visit this terrific network.

SHOPPING AND COOKING
California Dry Bean Board
www.calbeans.com/beanbasics.html
To learn more about cooking dried beans, check this out.

Penzeys Spices
800-741-7787
www.penzeys.com
This is an excellent source for high-quality spices, including sumac.

FOR MORE INFORMATION
Master Your Metabolism, Jillian Michaels

INDEX

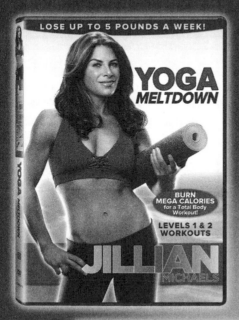
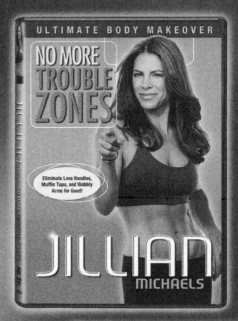
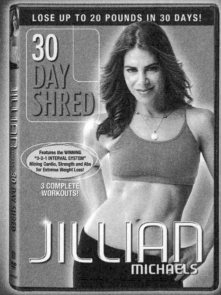
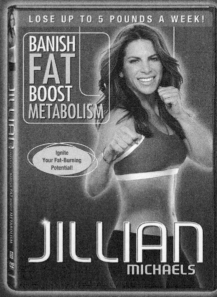

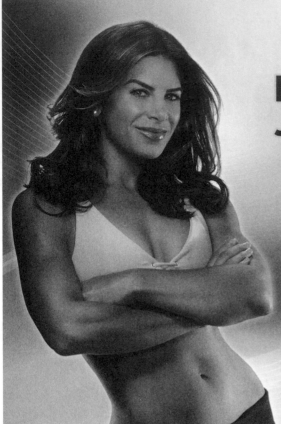